Audiologic Interpretation Across the Lifespan

DEBRA BUSACCO

Advanced Hearing Centers

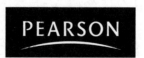

Boston   New York   San Francisco
Mexico City   Montreal   Toronto   London   Madrid   Munich   Paris
Hong Kong   Singapore   Tokyo   Cape Town   Sydney

Executive Editor and Publisher: *Stephen D. Dragin*
Editorial Assistant: *Anne Whittaker*
Vice President, Marketing and Sales Strategies: *Emily Williams Knight*
Vice President, Director of Marketing: *Quinn Perkson*
Production Editor: *Gregory Erb*
Editorial Production Service: *Walsh & Associates, Inc.*
Manufacturing Buyer: *Megan Cochran*
Electronic Composition: *Publishers' Design & Production Services*
Interior Design: *Publishers' Design & Production Services*
Cover Administrator: *Linda Knowles*

For related titles and support materials, visit our online catalog at
www.pearsonhighered.com.

Between the time website information is gathered and then published, it is not unusual for
some sites to have closed. Also, the transcription of URLs can result in typographical
errors. The publisher would appreciate notification where these errors occur so that they
may be corrected in subsequent editions.

Forms for audiograms in this book were used with permission from *Practical Forms for
Audiologists* copyright © 2003 American Speech-Language-Hearing Association, Rockville,
MD.

Printed in the United States of America

10 9 8 7 6 5 4 3 2 1 BRG 13 12 11 10 09

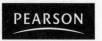
www.pearsonhighered.com

ISBN-10: 0-205-46398-3
ISBN-13: 978-0-205-46398-5

Dedication

To my sons, J.J. and Christian, who have taught me that patience and perseverance can make your dreams come true. I hope to instill in them a love of education, learning, and books.

To my deceased father, Albert, who taught me the value of education, hard work, and professional ethics and integrity. To my mother Lois, who has taught me as a professional woman the importance of balancing career and family. She has served as a wonderful role model for me over the years.

About the Author

Dr. Debra Busacco has more than 25 years of experience in the profession of audiology. She has conducted more than 55 national and international presentations. Dr. Busacco has numerous peer-reviewed publications. She has worked in a variety of settings including academia, clinical practices, and administration.

Contents

Preface   xi

PART 1   Audiometric Testing Principles and Audiogram Interpretation   1

Student Learning Outcomes   1

Population Demographics and the Incidence of Hearing Loss in the United States   1

Overview of Hearing Loss   2

    Types of Hearing Loss   3

        Conductive Hearing Loss   3

        Sensorineural Hearing Loss   3

        Mixed Hearing Loss   3

        Functional Hearing Loss   4

    Degree of Hearing Loss   4

    Audiometric Configuration   5

Components of the Audiologic Evaluation   6

    Case History Interview   6

    Otoscopic Examination   7

Pure Tone Air and Bone Conduction Audiometry   9

    Pure Tone Average   11

    Principles of Masking for Pure Tone Audiometry   11

        Masking for Pure Tone Air Conduction   12

        Masking for Pure Tone Bone Conduction   13

        Masking Problems   14

    Recording Pure Tone Audiometry Results   14

    Special Considerations in Pure Tone Audiometry   14

        Test Environment   14

        Earphone Selection   15

        Collapsed Ear Canals   15

        Test Instructions   15

Response Mode   *15*

Tactile Responses   *16*

Inconsistent Responses   *16*

Impacted Cerumen   *16*

Tinnitus Interference   *17*

Difficult-to-Test Patients   *18*

Functional Hearing Loss   18

Speech Audiometry   **19**

Speech Recognition Threshold/Speech Reception Threshold   19

Speech Detection Threshold/Speech Awareness Threshold   20

Word Recognition Score   20

Loudness Level   21

Most Comfortable Listening Level for Speech   *21*

Loudness Discomfort Level/Uncomfortable Listening Level for Speech   *22*

Masking for Speech Audiometry   22

Issues in Speech Audiometry   23

Test Environment   *23*

Presentation of Full-List Versus Half-List Speech Stimuli   *23*

Presentation Level of Speech Stimuli   *24*

Recorded Versus Monitored Live-Voice Testing   *24*

Use of Carrier Phrase   *24*

Test Condition   *25*

Response Mode   *25*

Soundfield Speech Audiometry   25

Testing Culturally and Linguistically Diverse Patients   26

Recording Speech Audiometry Results on the Audiogram   26

Objective Assessment of the Auditory System   **26**

Acoustic Immittance Battery   27

Tympanometry   *27*

Static Acoustic Compliance   *29*

Acoustic Reflex Thresholds   *30*

Acoustic Reflex Decay   *31*

Otoacoustic Emissions   31

Auditory Brainstem Response   32

Relationship Between Site of Lesion and ABR Results   *33*

Recording Audiological Data   **33**

Audiogram Interpretation Exercises   **35**

Clinical Enrichment Projects   63

Answers to Audiogram Interpretation Exercises   65

References   69

Recommended Readings   71

PART 2   **Audiologic Diagnosis and Management of Hearing Loss
             in the Pediatric Population**   **73**

Student Learning Outcomes   73

General Guidelines for Testing the Pediatric Population   73

Early Infant Hearing Detection Programs   75

Pediatric Audiologic Assessment   76

   Case History Interview   77

   Behavioral Testing of Children   77

      Behavioral Observation Audiometry   *80*

      Visual Reinforcement Audiometry   *80*

      Conditioned Orientation Reflex Audiometry   *81*

      Conditioned Play Audiometry   *81*

   Speech Audiometry Testing in Children   82

      Speech Detection/Speech Awareness Threshold in Children   *82*

      Speech Reception Threshold Testing in Children   *82*

      Word Recognition Testing in Children   *82*

   Objective Testing of the Pediatric Population   83

      Immittance Testing in Children   *84*

      Otoacoustic Emissions Testing in Children   *85*

      Auditory Brainstem Response Testing in Children   *85*

Special Considerations in the Pediatric Population   86

   Masking in Children   86

   Otitis Media in Children   86

   Unilateral Hearing Loss in Children   87

   Auditory Processing Disorders in Children   88

   Attention-Deficit/Hyperactivity Disorder and Auditory
   Processing Disorder   88

   Auditory Neuropathy in Children   88

   Functional Hearing Loss in Children   89

   Children with Physical and/or Mental Challenges   89

Intervention with Families from Culturally and Linguistically Diverse Backgrounds   90

Audiologic Intervention for Children with Hearing Loss   90

      Amplification Devices for Children 90

      Cochlear Implants for Children 91

      Educational Options for Children 91

Audiogram Interpretation Exercises **93**

Clinical Enrichment Projects **119**

Answers to Audiogram Interpretation Exercises **121**

References **125**

Recommended Readings **127**

PART 3   **Audiological Diagnosis and Management of Hearing Loss in the Older Adult Population** **129**

Student Learning Outcomes **129**

General Guidelines for Testing Older Adults **129**

Demographics of Older Adults in the United States **130**

Biological Changes Associated with Aging **131**

      Changes in the Nervous System 131

      Changes in the Visual System 132

      Changes in the Cardiovascular System 132

      Changes in the Renal System 132

      Changes in the Immune System 132

      Changes in the Somatosensory System 133

      Changes in Cognition 133

      Changes in the Vestibular System 133

      Changes in the Auditory System 134

Impacts of Aging **135**

      Impact of Aging on Audiometric Testing 135

      Impact of Aging on Speech Perception 135

      Impact of Aging on Otoacoustic Emissions 135

      Impact of Aging on the Auditory Brainstem Response 136

      Impact of Aging on the Middle Latency Response 136

      Impact of Aging on Auditory Late Responses (ALR) 136

Psychosocial Issues Related to Aging **136**

Special Considerations in Testing Older Adults **137**

      Audiologic Evaluation of Nursing Home Residents 137

      Audiologic Evaluation of Older Adults with Cognitive Impairment 138

Audiologic Rehabilitation Considerations in Older Adults **138**

Audiogram Interpretation Exercises   141

Clinical Enrichment Projects   163

Answers to Audiogram Interpretation Exercises   165

References   168

Recommended Readings   171

Glossary   **173**

Index   **179**

Preface

This book has been in the making for almost five years. It is my desire to provide students with an opportunity to engage in problem-based learning using a case study approach. The cases presented offer students a unique experience to make clinical decisions. Today's audiologists have numerous objective and behavioral tests that can be used as part of the audiology test battery. It is necessary that students understand the cost-effectiveness and sensitivity of each behavioral and objective test so as to recommend the most appropriate test protocol for each patient. Due to rising health care costs it is prudent to conduct only those audiologic tests that will provide the most diagnostic information about the site of lesion of the hearing loss. Hopefully, the cases presented will highlight the tests that provided the most information about the hearing loss.

This textbook is not intended to be a primary learning resource but as a supplement to any audiology textbook. It can be very useful for students in other disciplines including speech-language pathology, medicine, and education. The novice professional entering the clinical workplace will benefit from this practical resource depicting hearing loss related to a wide range of etiologies. The cases in each section provide a framework that can be used to build more advanced clinical cases. Faculty can use these cases to illustrate audiologic principles and help students gather information to aid in making accurate clinical decisions. The cases presented in this textbook can be used as individual or group learning activities. Student learning outcomes are presented for each Section. Faculty and clinical preceptors can add their own student learning outcomes and additional learning activities. The learning activities put forth in this book are designed to help students gain confidence in becoming "expert diagnosticians."

This book is divided into three parts. Part 1 focuses on a review of general audiologic information that can be applied to patients across the lifespan. Part 2 is a review of pediatric assessment. Part 3 provides a review of audiologic testing principles useful with adult and elderly patients. At the end of each section in Clinical Enrichment Projects, there are case studies for the population and issues addressed in that particular section. Students are provided with a series of questions along with possible answers. The questions are designed to help students integrate the audiologic data. Clinical Enrichment Projects are recommended at the end of each part. These projects are designed to help students go beyond the information presented in each part to further enhance their clinical knowledge and skills. Recommended Readings also are provided that include germane articles as well as professional position statements from the American Academy of Audiology (AAA) and the American Speech-Language-Hearing Association (ASHA).

ACKNOWLEDGMENTS

I would like to acknowledge my thanks to the many clinical supervisors, professors, and colleagues who taught me to constantly improve my audiologic diagnostic and management skills in order to provide quality care to patients with hearing loss and their families. I have learned immensely from each unique person.

To Steve Dragin for the encouragement and support necessary to take this manuscript from conception to book format. It has been a pleasure to be affiliated with Allyn and Bacon.

To the reviewers for their valuable feedback: Gerald T. Church, Central Michigan University; Bharti Katbama, Western Michigan University; Joseph Smaldino, Northern Illinois University; Linda Thibodeau, University of Texas at Dallas; Laura Ann Wilber, Northwestern University.

To Amanda Marchegiani for her extensive work as a student editor for this manuscript. To Kellye Carder and Dana Luzon for their review of the manuscript and their insight from a student's perspective. To future generations of students who will serve children and adults with hearing loss. My hope is that this book will further enhance your clinical skills and your confidence as you prepare to enter the dynamic and complex health care profession of audiology. I hope that you find this profession to be as fulfilling and as challenging a career as it has been for me.

Audiometric Testing Principles and Audiogram Interpretation

The purpose of this part is to provide a review of basic audiometric testing and audiogram interpretation. Students will interpret subjective and objective hearing tests including pure tone air and bone, speech audiometry, immittance battery, otoacoustic emissions (OAEs) and auditory brainstem response (ABR) results.

STUDENT LEARNING OUTCOMES

On completion of this part students will be able to:

1. Discuss demographics of hearing loss across the lifespan.
2. Describe the overall characteristics of hearing loss.
3. Describe the components of audiologic test procedures to diagnose hearing loss.
4. Interpret basic audiograms using pure tone, speech, and immittance data to determine the type and degree of hearing loss.
5. Interpret OAE data and ABR results.
6. Understand the impact of hearing loss on communication functioning.
7. Provide recommendations with rationales for audiologic intervention.

POPULATION DEMOGRAPHICS AND THE INCIDENCE OF HEARING LOSS IN THE UNITED STATES

The demographics of the U.S. population are changing dramatically. Individuals are living longer due to advancements in medical technology and an increased consciousness of the benefits of a healthy lifestyle. The population of the United States is aging. The mean age of women in this country is 76 years and the mean age for men is 72 years (U.S. Bureau of the Census, 2000). Both men and women are living longer and more productive lifestyles than ever in the history of the Unites States. Many neonates who at one time would have died due to medical complications at birth are surviving, albeit with disabilities such as hearing loss. Advances in genetic testing allow for the identification of genes that cause deafness. The implementation of state-mandated universal hearing screening programs has allowed for early identification and rehabilitation of hearing loss in infancy and childhood.

Hearing loss affects 1 in 10 individuals in the United States (Trychin & Busacco, 1991). Thirty-one million individuals have a hearing loss (Kochkin, 2005). Approximately 50 million individuals have tinnitus (American Tinnitus Association 2007). The number one reason for visits to the pediatrician is symptoms related to ear infections, with 90% of children experiencing at least one ear infection early in life (Northern & Downs, 2002). Age-related hearing loss affects about 40% to 50% of the U.S. population (Weinstein, 2000). As Americans age, the incidence of hearing loss will most likely increase so that persons with hearing loss who are age 65 and older will number 13 million by 2015. These estimates of hearing loss are probably an underestimation of the incidence of hearing loss across the age span, which most likely can be attributed to the lack of consistent hearing testing of children, adults, and elderly populations. In addition, oftentimes mild hearing loss or unilateral loss are undetected, and these individuals are not accounted for in the incidence data.

The U.S. population is growing in diversity. Audiologists providing hearing health care services need to be sensitive to the growing cultural and linguistic diversity of children and adults in the United States. In 2000, according to the 2000 U.S. census, 75.1% of the population white; 12.3% were black or African American; 3.6% were Asian or Pacific Islanders; 0.1% were American Indian, Eskimo, or Aleut; 0.2% were Native Hawaiian; and 2.4% were of two or more races. In terms of ethnicity, 87.5% were non-Hispanic and 12.5% were Hispanic (U.S. Bureau of the Census, 2000). Audiologists need to be aware of the impact of cultural and linguistic diversity on the provision of hearing health care services. Due to these demographic changes and the anticipated increase in hearing loss, the need for hearing and balance services will increase significantly over the next several decades, especially for patients who are from culturally diverse backgrounds (Battle, 2002).

OVERVIEW OF HEARING LOSS

The following information is a review of the characteristics of hearing loss. There are several types of hearing loss. The type of hearing loss will be determined by the location of damage (i.e., site of lesion) or pathology in the ear. Outer and/or middle ear medical pathologies result in a conductive hearing loss. Damage to the cochlea causes a sensorineural hearing loss, whereas pathology to the outer and/or middle and/or inner ear results is a mixed hearing loss. Damage to the VIII nerve or higher in the auditory central system results in a retrocochlear hearing loss. Hearing loss may be unilateral (i.e., on only one side) or bilateral, in which both ears are affected. Hearing loss that affects the outer ear up to the inner ear is a peripheral loss. Some individuals have auditory processing disorders (APD) resulting in central involvement. Two segments of the population at risk for auditory processing disorders are pediatric and elderly patients. Auditory processing disorders will be discussed further in Part 2 and Part 3.

Types of Hearing Loss

The following is an overview of the types of hearing loss and some common characteristics of communication problems associated with each type.

Conductive hearing loss. A conductive hearing loss results from damage to the outer and/or middle ear. This type of hearing loss causes decrease in loudness. In a conductive loss, there is a hearing impairment for air conduction with normal bone conduction. Most individuals will report minimal problems with the clarity of speech as long as acoustic stimuli are presented at a level that is sufficiently loud. Conductive hearing loss typically does not exceed 60 dB HL (decibels hearing level). For the majority of conductive pathologies, there is some type of medical and/or surgical intervention that will restore hearing sensitivity to near or within normal limits. In those cases in which medical treatment is not a viable option, patients can benefit from amplification devices because they make sounds louder, which overcomes the loss of intensity and makes speech intelligible.

Sensorineural hearing loss. Sensorineural hearing loss can be either cochlear or retrocochlear (i.e., with VIII nerve involvement) or both. This type of hearing loss is characterized by a loss of clarity of speech. There is a hearing loss for both air and bone conduction, and thresholds are within 10 dB HL of one another. The degree of hearing loss may range from mild to profound. The audiometric contour can take on a variety of configurations. For this type of hearing loss, there is usually no medical or surgical intervention to restore hearing sensitivity to within normal limits. Otologic problems that accompany sensorineural hearing loss may include tinnitus, balance problems, and physiological recruitment. Approximately 50% of individuals with sensorineural hearing loss also experience tinnitus (Tyler, 2000). Several inner ear conditions such as labyrinthitis, Lyme disease, and Ménière's disease can result in dizziness or vertigo for which there may be some medication to relieve symptoms. Most patients with sensorineural hearing loss are good candidates for audiologic rehabilitation including amplification, cochlear implantation, communication strategies training, speechreading, and auditory training. In cases of retrocochlear hearing loss due to a VIII nerve tumor, there may be surgical intervention to remove the tumor for life-saving purposes. The patient's hearing may be saved or it may be destroyed depending on the size and location of the tumor. A VIII tumor is rare, with only 5% of individuals affected by this condition (Tyler, 2000). The majority of patients who are hard of hearing and deaf have sensorineural hearing loss that is cochlear in origin.

Mixed hearing loss. A mixed hearing loss causes a hearing loss for both air and bone conduction with a greater than 15 dB HL difference between these thresholds. Air-bone gaps are present, with air conduction thresholds being poorer than bone conduction thresholds. Site of lesion is the outer and/or middle and inner ear. The conductive portion of the hearing loss may be medically treatable, but the sensorineural portion will remain. An example of a mixed hearing loss might be one caused by an impacted cerumen and presbycusis. The cerumen can be removed; however, the presbycusic hearing loss remains after medical intervention.

Functional hearing loss. A small portion of an audiologist's caseload will comprise children and adults who feign or pretend to have a hearing loss. There are a variety of terms used to describe when an individual exaggerates having a hearing loss. Some of the terms are *functional*, *nonorganic*, and *malingering* hearing loss. The term that will be used in this textbook is *functional hearing loss*. The individual feigning the hearing loss may have an underlying organic hearing loss, but the degree of loss and its impact on communication function are exaggerated. Some of the reasons an individual may pretend to have a hearing loss are related to compensation for insurance purposes or results of a psychological trauma. Oftentimes, in children, a functional hearing loss is related to a psychological event such as parental divorce, abuse, or academic difficulties. Although functional hearing loss is rare, it should be investigated if audiometric inconsistencies are present or a patient's behavior is suspect during the test session.

The type of hearing loss will determine the rehabilitation options as well as the impact on communication abilities. The impact of a hearing loss on an individual will vary depending on his or her physical condition, psychosocial status, and other variables that will be addressed later in this textbook.

Degree of Hearing Loss

In addition to the classification of hearing loss based on site of lesion in the auditory system, it is also described based on degree of loss. Table 1.1 illustrates a classification system of degree of hearing loss for children and adults (Stach,

TABLE 1.1 Classification of Degree of Hearing Loss for Children and Adults

	Degree of Hearing Loss (dB HL)	
Degree	**Children**	**Adults**
Normal	10–15	10–25
Slight	16–25	Not a category
Mild	26–40	26–40
Moderate	41–55	41–55
Moderately Severe	56–70	56–70
Severe	71–90	71–90
Profound	>90	>90

Adapted from Stach, B. (1999). *Clinical audiology: An introduction.* San Diego: Singular.

1999). Audiologists tend to describe the degree of hearing loss based on the three-frequency pure tone average (PTA), which is the average air conduction thresholds at 500 Hz, 1000 Hz, and 2000 Hz in each ear. It is helpful to describe the degree of hearing loss on a frequency-by-frequency basis so as to understand its impact on speech understanding ability across the frequency range.

Audiometric Configuration

It is critical for pure tone data to be interpreted based on the audiometric configuration of the hearing loss. Table 1.2 provides a general classification system for describing the overall audiometric contour of the audiogram (Stach, 1999). The information presented in Table 1.2 should be used as guideline to describe the overall contour of the hearing loss. Most hearing loss will not fit into one clear-cut contour. It is recommended that the audiologist describe the audiometric contour of the hearing loss across the frequency range so as to gain an understanding of the possible impact on speech understanding.

This section provided a review of audiogram interpretation to determine the type, degree, and audiometric configuration of the hearing loss. This information will be used by the audiologist to gain an understanding of the communication challenges an individual may experience in a variety of listening environments. Typically, individuals with a mild-to-severe hearing loss are considered to be hard of hearing. Those with a severe-to-profound hearing loss are classified as audiologically deaf. The psychological implications of the hearing loss are different for individuals who are hard of hearing as compared to those who are deaf. The audiologic recommendations made will be based on not only the hearing loss but also on an individual's attitude and motivation to be involved in the audiologic rehabilitation process.

TABLE 1.2   Classification of Audiometric Configuration

Flat	Thresholds are within 20 dB HL of each other across the frequency range.
Rising	Thresholds for low frequencies are at least 20 dB poorer than for high frequencies.
Sloping	Thresholds for higher frequencies are at least 20 dB poorer than for lower frequencies.
Low-Frequency	Hearing loss only in the low frequencies.
High-Frequency	Hearing loss only in the high frequencies.
Precipitously Sloping	Steeply sloping high-frequency hearing loss with 20 dB or greater loss per octave.
Miscellaneous	Does not fit any of the above categories.

Adapted from Stach, B. (1999). *Clinical audiology: An introduction.* San Diego: Singular.

COMPONENTS OF THE AUDIOLOGIC EVALUATION

The following is an overview of the components of the basic audiologic evaluation.

Case History Interview

One of the most critical components of the evaluation process is taking a comprehensive case history. The information gleaned from a good case history can provide audiologists and medical professionals with the information necessary to diagnose the hearing loss. The case history should provide information about general health status and educational, vocational, and social implications related to the patient's hearing loss. Additional areas will be included based on the chronological and developmental age of the patient. The questions will vary depending on whether the patient is a child, adult, or elderly. Every clinic should have a separate case history form for each aforementioned population. If there is a large proportion of patients for whom English is a second language (ESL), then the case history interview should be conducted in their native languages so as to obtain accurate information. This can be accomplished through a professional interpreter. Hopefully, more audiologists will be multilingual in the future, especially if they are providing hearing health care services on a regular basis to a specific group of culturally and linguistically diverse patients.

It is critical for students to understand that taking a good case history is a combined art and science. Initially, most students will ask the patient every question that is on the case history form. Over time, students need to be able to listen to the patient's and/or family's concerns and move freely from question to question based on the patient's responses, eliminating nonrelevant items from the case history interview.

The case history form can be given to the patient prior to the audiology appointment through either mail or email. The audiologist should review the pertinent information with the patient during the initial visit. It is imperative that the case history information be reviewed with the patient in a face-to-face manner for several reasons. First, most likely during the case history interview, the patient will expand on answers provided in writing. Second, the case history interview can be an opportunity for the audiologist to gain insight into the patient's personality and communication style. Third, this exchange of information will be the beginning of the professional rapport between the patient and family or significant other(s) and the audiologist.

During the case history interview, the audiologist should demonstrate empathy for the patient's situation. This is especially imperative when dealing with the pediatric population and the reactions of the family or significant other(s). The clinician should realize that it has taken the majority of patients a long time to seek an evaluation, especially older adults and those individuals who are in denial. The audiologist should view the case history interview as the first step in the process of developing a trusting relationship with the patient and family or significant other(s).

The components of a general case history should include demographic and identifying information, concern about hearing and balance problems, previous audiologic and otolaryngology histories, medical background, and medication history. Additional information will be added depending on the population for whom the case history is designed. For example, with the pediatric population, there should be extensive questions related to pregnancy history, infants' hearing screening results, and developmental milestones. In the elderly population, there is a need to obtain information about medications, cognitive status, and other sensory losses (e.g., vision). The information obtained from a thorough case history can be valuable in helping the audiologist determine which tests to conduct, the site of lesion, and the possible etiology of the hearing loss.

Sample case histories of adults and children are provided in the Audiogram Interpretation Exercises at the end of the appropriate part of this textbook. The adult case history intake form can be modified for the elderly population. Each case presented in this textbook is accompanied by pertinent history information to assist the student in putting this information together with audiologic test results. When counseling a patient about the diagnostic findings, the audiologist should revert back to the case history information to help the patient understand the relationship between the hearing and/or balance complaints and the audiologic findings.

A sample adult case history developed by ASHA is included in Figure 1.1. This case history can serve as a guideline for interviewing adults and can be modified for the elderly population.

The pediatric case history is included in Part 2. Students are encouraged to use the case history information to diagnose the patient's hearing loss and make appropriate audiologic rehabilitation recommendations.

Otoscopic Examination

Prior to starting the audiologic testing, an otoscopic examination is necessary to visualize the external ear canal and the tympanic membrane. An otoscope can range from a simple handheld device to a more sophisticated video-otoscope that can take photographs of the external ear. An otoscope allows for light illumination and magnification to assess whether there is inflammation, infection, impacted cerumen, and/or other pathologies in the external ear canal or pathology of the tympanic membrane. If an otologic pathology is suspected, then the patient should be referred for an otology examination. When the patient has impacted cerumen and the audiologist is trained in removing it, then this procedure should be done prior to conducting the hearing evaluation. If impacted cerumen is present when doing the examination, then audiologic test results may be compromised, as there can be a 20 dB HL–40 dB HL conductive hearing loss resulting in false air-bone gaps. It is imperative that the major landmarks, including the cone of light, possibly the umbo, and the pearly gray translucent color of the tympanic membrane, are present. Absence of these landmarks may suggest an abnormal examination, and medical referral should be made.

Practitioner Name or Practice
Address
City, State Zipcode
Phone Number – Fax Number
Web site – E-mail Address

Adult Case History

Name:	
Date:	

1. Do you feel that you are experiencing a hearing problem? ☐Yes ☐No

   If yes, how long have you been aware of the problem?

2. Do you feel that one ear is better than the other? ☐Yes ☐No

   If so, which is your better ear? ☐Right ☐Left

3. In what listening situations do you have difficulty hearing? (i.e., one-on-one

   conversations, groups, work, church, restaurants, TV, theaters, etc.)

4. Have you ever worn a hearing aid? ☐Yes ☐No

   If yes, for how long?

5. Have you ever had medical treatment or surgery for ear problems? ☐Yes ☐No

6. Have you had any recent ear pain or drainage? ☐Yes ☐No

7. Do you have any allergies? ☐Yes ☐No

8. Do you ever experience noises in your ears? ☐Yes ☐No

   (i.e., ringing, buzzing, etc.)

9. Have you experienced dizziness or loss of balance within the

   last 90 days that you cannot relate to a specific cause? ☐Yes ☐No

FIGURE 1.1 ASHA Case History

American Speech-Language-Hearing Association (ASHA) (2003), *Practical Forms for Audiologists.* Rockville, MD.

10. Have you ever experienced a serious head injury? ☐Yes ☐No

11. How would you describe your general health? ☐Good ☐Average ☐Fair ☐Poor

12. Are you currently taking any medications? ☐Yes ☐No

   If so, please list what conditions they are for:

13. Have you ever had a serious illness that may have affected your hearing?

   (i.e., scarlet fever, meningitis, mumps, etc.) ☐Yes ☐No

14. Have you ever been exposed to high levels of sound? (i.e., farm equipment,

   power tools, lawn movers, chain saws, snow blowers, industrial machinery,

   firearms, etc.) ☐Yes ☐No

15. Does anyone in your family have a hearing loss? ☐Yes ☐No

   If so, what caused it?

16. Do you have any other significant health problems or handicaps? ☐Yes ☐No

17. Do you have any speech, language, or voice problems? ☐Yes ☐No

18. What questions or problems would you like help with today?

FIGURE 1.1 Continued

PURE TONE AIR AND BONE CONDUCTION AUDIOMETRY

The basic audiologic tests used to determine the type, degree, and audiometric configuration are pure tone air and bone conduction audiometry. Pure tone audiometry is used to establish hearing threshold levels. Hearing threshold level is defined as the lowest intensity level that a pure tone can be heard 50% of the time. Pure tone audiometry is a conventional behavioral test that requires a response from the patient. Results of pure tone air and bone conduction testing are recorded on the audiogram. Figure 1.2 is a sample audiogram from ASHA (2003). This audiogram will be used throughout this textbook.

The ordinate of the audiogram is hearing level in dBHL ranging from the lowest intensity of –10 dBHL to the highest intensity of 120 dBHL. The horizontal scale, or abscissa, represents the frequency of the pure tone ranging from a low frequency of 125 Hz to a high frequency of 8000 Hz. Typically, pure tone air conduction thresholds are measured at octaves from 250 Hz to 8000 Hz and

NAME:_____   AGE/DATE OF BIRTH: _____

REFERRED BY: _____   MEDICAL RECORD #: _____

TEST INTERVAL: _____   DATE OF TEST: _____

PURE TONE AUDIOMETRY (RE: ANSI 1996)

KEY:

LEFT	STIMULUS	RIGHT
X	AIR	O
□	AIR - MASK	△
>	BONE	<
]	BONE - MASK	[
↘	NO RESPONSE	↙
L	AIDED SOUND FIELD	R
	SOUND FIELD = **S**	

TEST TYPE
- STANDARD CAE
- PLAY
- COR/VRA
- BOA

TRANSDUCER
- INSERT
- CIRCUMAURAL
- SOUND FIELD

RELIABILITY
- EXCELLENT
- GOOD
- FAIR
- POOR

BOOTH
- #1
- #2 (PEDS)
- #3
- #4 COCH IMPLANT

TYMPANOMETRY (226 Hz)

EAR	LEFT	RIGHT
STATIC ADMITTANCE (mm H$_2$O)		
TYMP PEAK PRESSURE (DaPa)		
TYMP WIDTH (DaPa)		
EAR CANAL VOLUME cm^3		

LEFT   RIGHT

Admittance

Pressure   Pressure

CONTRA	.5k Hz	1k Hz	2k Hz	4k Hz	IPSI	.5k Hz	1k Hz	2k Hz	4k Hz
Right (AD) (phone ear)					AD (probe ear)				
Left (AS) (phone ear)					AS (probe ear)				

MIDDLE EAR ANALYZER _____

SPEECH AUDIOMETRY

	PTA	SRT/ SAT	Speech Recognition	Speech Recognition	MCL	UCL
RIGHT (AD)						
			%	%		
Masking						
LEFT (AS)						
			%	%		
Masking						

MLV □	CD/tape □	W-22 □	WIPI □	PBK □	SPECIAL:		SPECIAL:
SOUND FIELD			%		%		
RIGHT AIDED			%		%		
LEFT AIDED			%		%		
BINAURAL			%		%		

OTOACOUSTIC EMISSIONS (OAEs)

EMISSION TYPE USED	TEST TYPE PERFORMED
Transient	OAE Complete
Distortion Product	OAE Screening
OAE results:	
Right Ear	
Left Ear	

OAE UNIT _____

HEARING AID INFORMATION

RIGHT AID: _____

LEFT AID: _____

OTOSCOPY: _____

HISTORY/IMPRESSIONS/RECOMMENDATIONS: _____

_____

_____

_____

_____

_____

AUDIOLOGIST:_____   ASSISTANT:_____   AUDIOMETER:_____

FIGURE 1.2 ASHA Audiogram

American Speech-Language-Hearing Association (ASHA). (2003), *Practical Forms for Audiologists.* Rockville, MD: Author.

PART 1   Audiometric Testing Principles and Audiogram Interpretation

bone conduction thresholds are measured at octaves from 500 Hz to 4000 Hz. Interoctave frequencies are tested when there is a 20 dB HL difference between two octaves. For example, if the pure tone threshold is 40 dB HL at 500 Hz and 60 dB HL at 1000 Hz, then the interoctave of 750 Hz should be tested. The testing of interoctave frequencies will provide more information about the audiometric contour and the potential impact of hearing loss on communication abilities.

Pure Tone Average

The pure tone average (PTA) refers to the average air conduction thresholds at 500 Hz, 1000 Hz, and 2000 Hz. There is a good correlation between the mean of these three thresholds and the speech reception threshold (SRT). If there is a significant difference among these three thresholds, then the best two frequencies of the three frequencies should be used to calculate the PTA. The two-frequency pure tone average, referred to as Fletcher's Average, will be in better agreement with the SRT than the three-frequency pure tone average in steeply sloping audiograms (Fletcher, 1950). The relationship between the PTA and SRT serves as a reliability check of the patient's responses. These two diagnostics measurements should be within ±5 dB HL. If there is no agreement, then the test results may not be reliable, and the possible reason(s) for inconsistent responses should be determined. One reason for inconsistencies may be false positive or false negative responses. If the patient responds when no acoustic stimulus is presented, then this is considered to be a false positive response. If the patient does not respond when an acoustic stimulus is presented, then this is considered to be a false negative response. False positive and false negative responses will impact on inter- and intratest reliability of the audiologic data.

Principles of Masking for Pure Tone Audiometry

At times, depending on the type and severity of the hearing loss, it may be necessary to keep the nontest ear from participating in the test situation due to the phenomenon known as cross-hearing. Cross-hearing occurs when a tone of sufficient intensity introduced into the test ear crosses over to the nontest ear via bone conduction or sound leakage from the earphones. The result is that the patient will think the tone is in the test ear and will provide a false positive response, resulting in an inaccurate threshold. Cross-hearing can be eliminated by introducing masking noise into the nontest ear to shift the hearing thresholds to a poorer level so that cross hearing is eliminated. Masking can be done for both air and bone conduction testing. One rule is that whenever masking is necessary for air conduction, it is also necessary to mask for bone conduction. However, it may be necessary to mask for bone conduction but not air conduction. Although a variety of formulae exist to help determine the appropriate masking level, it is critical to understand the underlying principles of masking in order to make correct clinical decisions about the type and degree of hearing loss. If errors are made when masking, then there may be erroneous test results, and a misdiagnosis can occur.

Masking for pure tone air conduction.   Masking is necessary for air conduction testing when a 40 dB HL difference exists between air conduction thresholds in the test ear and bone conduction thresholds in the nontest ear. Masking for bone conduction is necessary when there is a 10 dB HL or greater difference between the air and bone conduction thresholds at a particular frequency. If the pure tone air or bone signal is of sufficient magnitude so that it can cross over to the nontest ear, then masking needs to be done. When the test ear is not isolated through masking erroneous hearing, thresholds will be obtained and a misdiagnosis of the type and degree of hearing loss will result.

When masking, the key concept to understand is that it is necessary to shift the bone conduction threshold of the nontest ear at the test frequency so that the patient will not hear the tone in the nontest ear. In order to shift the bone conduction threshold, the air conduction threshold also needs to be shifted to a poorer hearing level. Air and bone conduction thresholds are shifted by the same amount, but the thresholds may be shifted to different hearing levels. Yacullo (1996) stated that effective masking (EM) is defined as the hearing level in decibels to which the threshold is shifted by a given noise level. For example, at 1000 Hz, the air conduction threshold in the good ear is 20 dB HL, and the air conduction threshold is 65 dB HL in the poorer ear. The bone conduction threshold is 15 dB HL and assumed to be the response of the good ear. If a signal of 65 dB HL is presented using supra-aural earphones with an inter aural attenuation value of 40 dB HL, then 25 dB HL of sound crosses over to the nontest ear. Given that the air conduction threshold is 20 dB HL, the test tone can be heard in the nontest ear and the patient will respond. In order to keep the nontest ear from participating in the test, masking noise must be put into the nontest ear in order to shift the air and bone conduction thresholds to a poorer level so that the sound intensity crossing over will not be heard and accurate thresholds are obtained. Consequently, the air conduction thresholds obtained will be accurate.

The type of masking noise used for pure tone audiometry is narrowband noise. Fletcher and Munson (1937) showed that the use of a narrow band of noise centered around the frequency provided the best masker for the pure tone stimulus. For more information about masking refer to Yacullo (1996).

Masking is one of the most difficult concepts for students and new clinicians to master. The most likely reason for this difficulty is the sequential and hierarchical decisions that need to be made by the clinician in a short period of time during the testing session. It is recommended that students spend time studying the concepts of masking using clinical cases and, possibly, simulated software programs to help them gain confidence in making clinical masking decisions. The following are the decisions that need to be made when determining if masking is necessary for pure tone air and bone conduction audiometry:

1. Is masking necessary for air conduction?
2. Is masking necessary for bone conduction?

3. If yes, which ear needs to be masked so that it will not participate in the testing situation?

4. At which frequencies does masking need to be done for air conduction, bone conduction, or both?

5. How much noise needs to be delivered to the nontest ear at each frequency?

6. When the noise is introduced into the nontest ear, to what hearing levels are air and bone conduction thresholds being shifted at each frequency?

Several formulae have been put forth to determine the initial masking level for the noise in the nontest ear. According to Martin and Clark (2005), the formula used to determine the initial masking level for air conduction (AC) is as follows:

AC nte (air conduction threshold in the nontest ear) + 10 dBHL (safety factor) = initial masking level in the nontest ear

Masking for pure tone bone conduction. When determining the initial masking level for bone conduction, it is necessary to include the occlusion effect in the formula. The occlusion effect is defined as an improvement in bone conduction thresholds at 500 Hz and 1000 Hz that occurs as a result of placing an earphone over the nontest ear when the bone conduction oscillator is placed on the mastoid. Typically, there is no occlusion effect for the high frequencies of 2000 Hz and 4000 Hz. The amount of occlusion effect is calculated by comparing bone conduction thresholds without the earphone over the nontest ear to bone conduction thresholds obtained with an earphone over the test ear. The amount of occlusion effect varies by frequency and across individuals. The amount of occlusion effect must be included when calculating the initial masking level.

According to Martin and Clark (2005), the formula used to determine the initial masking level for bone conduction (BC) is as follows:

AC nte (air conduction threshold in the nontest ear) + OC (occlusion effect) + 10 dB HL (safety factor) = initial masking level in the nontest ear

Once the initial masking level is attained, the next step is to establish the threshold in the test ear. Typically, this is done using the Hood Plateau (Katz, 2002). Whenever the threshold in the test ear shifts by 5 dB HL, the masking noise is increased by 10 dB HL. This procedure is followed until a 20 dB HL range is achieved when the hearing threshold in the test ear does not shift despite an increase in masking noise. This 20 dB HL range is known as the Hood Plateau. When the threshold is maintained for the 20 dB HL plateau, then the true threshold of the test ear has been obtained. Both the unmasked and masked air and bone conduction thresholds are recorded on the audiogram as well as the masking levels of noise used to establish the Hood Plateau at each frequency tested (DeBonis & Donohue, 2006).

Masking problems.   Two problems that can occur when masking are (1) under-masking and (2) overmasking. These issues can result in not attaining effective masking levels and in erroneous hearing threshold levels.

Undermasking.   In cases of undermasking, erroneous thresholds are obtained as a result of not presenting enough masking noise to the nontest ear. Conse-quently, cross-hearing occurs and the tone is heard in the nontest ear so the true thresholds of the test ear are not obtained. In the majority of clinical cases, undermasking is a more prevalent phenomenon than overmasking, especially if students are not analyzing the amount of threshold shift that is occurring when the masking noise is introduced at different intensity levels.

Overmasking.   Overmasking results when there is too much noise put into the nontest ear. The result is that the noise crosses over from the nontest ear to the test ear, thereby obliterating the testing tone. In cases of overmasking, the patient's threshold will be artificially elevated (i.e., poorer) as the noise obliter-ates the tone presented at or near the true hearing threshold level.

Recording Pure Tone Audiometry Results

The audiogram that will be used throughout this book has been put forth by the American Speech-Language-Hearing Association (2003). Unmasked air con-duction thresholds are depicted by "O" for the right ear and "X" for the left ear. Masked air conduction thresholds are depicted by "Δ" for the right ear and "□" for the left ear. Unmasked bone conduction thresholds are illustrated using a carat opening to the right "<" for placement of the oscillator on the right mas-toid and a carat with the opening to the left ">" for placement on the left mas-toid. Masked bone conduction thresholds are indicated by a "[" for the right ear and a "]"for the left ear. No response at the maximum power output of the audiometer for air and bone conduction thresholds is depicted by the appropri-ate symbol with an attached arrow ⟋ ⤬ ⟨⟍ ⟍⟩. When recording soundfield results the symbol "S" is used. Several abbreviations may also be noted on the audiogram, including "CNT" for "could not test" and "DNT" for "did not test." Any additional symbols or abbreviations used that are not in the ASHA legend should be noted on the audiogram.

Special Considerations in Pure Tone Audiometry

Audiologists need to be aware of several issues that can impact pure tone air and bone conduction thresholds. Each issue is described and solutions are presented to better ensure that reliable and valid pure tone thresholds are obtained.

Test environment.   The test environment in which pure tone audiometry is con-ducted should meet the current Standards for Allowable Ambient Noise Levels of the American National Standards Institute (ANSI, 1999). All equipment should meet the manufacturer's specifications and ANSI 1996 Standards for Audiometers.

Earphone selection.   There are several different earphones available for hearing testing. These include TDH-39, TDH-49, and TDH-50 supra-aural earphones and insert earphones. Whenever possible, insert earphones should be used over supra-aural earphones. The benefits of insert earphones include better comfort for the patient; elimination of collapsed ear canals; reduction in the level of ambient noise levels; greater interaural attenuation values up to 70 dB HL, which eliminates the need for masking; and the ability to test each ear independently. More clinics across the country are using insert earphones on a routine basis due to the aforementioned associated benefits, especially with the pediatric population. Most infants and children will tolerate insert earphones as compared to supra-aural earphones, thereby allowing the audiologist to obtain test information on each ear.

Collapsed ear canals.   Collapsed ear canals are the result of pressure from the headband and the supra-aural earphones on the pinnae, resulting in false air-bone gaps that simulate a conductive hearing loss. This temporary condition is most prevalent in pediatric and elderly patients due to the lack of cartilage of the pinnae, causing closure of the orifice of the external auditory canal. Typically, air-bone gaps will be present at high frequencies; however, any frequency can be affected. Collapsed ear canals should be suspected when the case history and immittance data do not support the presence of either a conductive or mixed hearing loss.

Test instructions.   The instructions provided to a patient are critical in terms of the response that can be expected. The criteria used by the patient will be based on the instructions provided for a particular test. Some patients will use conservative response criteria that can result in higher-than-expected hearing thresholds. Other patients will be more liberal in responding, possibly resulting in more false positive responses. Audiologists need to keep instructions clear and concise by telling the patient the type of acoustic stimuli that will be presented and expected responses and encourage guessing when the stimulus is at or near threshold. If the patient reports tinnitus, it may be necessary to use a pulsed tone to assist the patient in differentiating the pure tone stimulus from the tinnitus. It is critical that the audiologist encourage the patient to respond to the pure tone stimuli even if the tones are very soft when they are at or near threshold. Test instructions should be simple, clear, and concise to eliminate testing or patient artifacts that would result in nonvalid test data.

Response mode.   There are a variety of responses patients can use to indicate that an acoustic stimulus was detected. The most common response is raising a hand or pressing a button when a tone is detected. A second common response that can be used with patients who are cognitively alert is saying "yes" when a stimulus is detected. Giving a verbal response tends to be faster than using the hand-raising technique for most adults, especially the elderly population. The goal in determining the most appropriate response mode is to ensure that the patient's responses are consistent throughout the test session. In order to assess reliability, it is critical to retest the patient's air conduction threshold at 1000 Hz for each ear. The 1000 Hz test/retest reliability of the air conduction thresholds should be within +/–5 dB HL. If this agreement does not exist, then the patient should be reinstructed and retested to obtain accurate responses.

Some other modifications that can be made for pure tone testing for a non-verbal patient include augmentative and alternative communication devices (AAC), eye blinking, foot tapping, or nodding of the head in response to auditory stimuli. The response mode selected will be determined by the communication and cognitive abilities of each patient. The types of responses that can be expected from pediatric patients are addressed in Part 2, and those expected from older adults are provided in Part 3.

Tactile responses.   One problem that can arise in air and bone conduction testing at high intensity levels is tactile or vibratory responses. Vibratory responses typically are present in the low frequencies (e.g., 250–500 Hz), especially if the tones are being presented at the maximum power output of the audiometer. Tactile bone conduction thresholds should be suspected in cases of severe-to-profound hearing loss, especially in the low frequencies. Oftentimes, the patient will report "feeling" the tone rather than "hearing" it. The tones that are "felt" are not the true thresholds of the patient. Patients should be instructed to notify the audiologist when the auditory stimuli is felt rather than heard.

Inconsistent responses.   It is critical that a patient's responses during pure tone testing are consistent. Consistent responses mean that the test results are likely to be reliable and valid. Unreliable responses may include false positive and false negative responses as defined earlier. Inconsistent responses may be the results of the patient's lack of understanding test instructions or feigning a hearing loss. Test/retest reliability at 1000 Hz for pure tone thresholds is an indicator of good intratest reliability. The test/retest thresholds should be within ±5 dB HL of each other. An example intertest of reliability is evaluating the relationship between the pure tone average (PTA) and the speech recognition threshold (SRT). This relationship should be within ±5 dB HL. Another intertest reliability measure includes the comparison of acoustic reflex thresholds and pure tone thresholds to assess their relationship to each other.

Some individuals, especially those with cognitive impairment, may never be able to provide consistent responses, especially to pure tone stimuli. Whenever there are inconsistent responses, the audiologist should try to determine the reason(s) for the inconsistency so that accurate thresholds can be obtained. For individuals who exhibit inconsistent responses, hearing status can be determined using a combination of subjective and objective tests including speech, otoacoustic emissions, and auditory brainstem response measurements.

Impacted cerumen.   In most individuals, cerumen moves out of the ear canal on its own (Ballachanda, 1995). In some individuals there is an accumulation of cerumen that forms in the ear canal and can cause occlusion. Depending upon the amount of occlusion, a conductive hearing loss may be present. Incidence of excessive impacted cerumen in the general population is 2–6%; in the pediatric population, about 10%; and in the elderly population it may be as high as 34% (Ballachanda, 1995). Impacted cerumen may result in a sudden hearing loss; 100% occlusion may cause tinnitus, feeling of blockage, hearing loss, and increased likelihood of infection.

Impacted cerumen tends to be common in the pediatric population due to the small size of the ear canals. A large percentage of older adults also will have impacted cerumen due to age-related changes in the ceruminous and sebaceous glands (Ballachanda, 1995). The occlusion of the ear canal can result in a conductive hearing loss that can be as great as 20–40 dB HL. The treatment is removal of the cerumen. Once the cerumen is removed, the conductive hearing loss is ameliorated. Impacted cerumen can cause a delay in audiologic service delivery by weeks and, in some cases, months, especially when dealing with the nursing home population. A cerumen removal protocol should be in place in every test setting so as not to delay hearing health care services. Many audiologists have been trained in cerumen removal, thereby eliminating the need for referral and delayed follow-up care. Although cerumen management is in the scope of practice for audiologists, typically there is no reimbursement, and state licensure statutes will determine if audiologists are allowed to remove cerumen.

Tinnitus interference. Oftentimes, individuals with hearing loss experience a ringing sound in the ear(s) and/or head known as tinnitus. It has been estimated that approximately 12 million individuals report tinnitus either on a consistent or intermittent basis (American Tinnitus Association, 2007). Tinnitus has been described in a variety of ways including ringing, buzzing, roaring, hissing, crackling, and whooshing. Tinnitus can range being from an annoyance to very debilitating. In its severest cases, it can be linked to reduced quality of life, depression, and suicidal thoughts. Tinnitus can become a major source of stress in one's life and can interfere with activities of daily living. It may result in lack of concentration, reduced sleep, and withdrawl from social activities that were once meaningful. The cause of tinnitus in most cases is unknown. It may be related to damage in the peripheral and/or central auditory systems. Tinnitus may be present on either a continuous or intermittent basis. The loudness of the tinnitus may change over time (e.g., daily to weekly), especially in cases of Ménière's disease, high blood pressure, or stress. Whenever tinnitus is present, otologic, audiologic, and medical evaluations must be conducted to determine its possible etiology and treatment. When a patient reports that the tinnitus is debilitating and impacting on his or her quality of life, there should be a referral to an audiologist, ear, nose, and throat (ENT) physician, and possibly a psychologist who specializes in tinnitus, as this condition can impact audiologic recommendations and patient management.

It is critical to know whether the patient's tinnitus may interfere with detection of pure tones during the hearing evaluation. If the tinnitus and the pure tones have similar acoustic characteristics (e.g., intensity and frequency), then the patient may not be able to differentiate the tone from the tinnitus. Oftentimes, when the tinnitus interferes with detecting a tone, the patient will exhibit either false negative or false positive responses. This can be remediated by pulsing the pure tone stimuli to make them more detectable, especially when the pure tone is at or near the patient's auditory threshold.

Difficult-to-test patients. There will be some patients for whom it will be difficult to conduct conventional pure tone audiometry. Some difficult-to-test patients may include young children and individuals with developmental disabilities, emotional disorders, cognitive impairment, and/or neurological disorders. In such cases, the audiologist needs to be creative in combining both behavioral and objective tests to obtain as much information as possible about the patient's hearing status. Special considerations in evaluating difficult-to-test patients will be included in other parts of this textbook.

In summary, these aforementioned problems can impact pure tone audiometry and need to be considered when conducting pure tone testing. Despite the numerous advances in audiologic testing such as OAEs and auditory evoked potentials (AEPs), the basic audiologic evaluation is the backbone of the diagnosis test battery. Pure tone audiometry should not be substituted by objective assessments. A combination of behavioral and electrophysiological assessments is recommended as a cross-check of the patient's test results (Jerger & Hayes, 1976).

Functional Hearing Loss

In functional hearing loss, there is usually a discrepancy or inconsistency between audiologic test results, especially in the relationship between pure tone and speech data. A common finding is a lack of agreement between the PTA and SRT. In most cases, the SRT is better than the PTA. Oftentimes, during SRT testing, the patient will give half-word responses for spondees. This should not occur, as spondee words have equal stress on each syllable; therefore the entire spondee word should be heard. When examining word recognition results, the patient will perform better than expected as compared to the pure tone audiometry results. For example, an individual with a significant sensorineural hearing loss may exhibit excellent word recognition scores when testing at levels lower or equal to those that have been provided. Although it is difficult to predict word recognition scores from pure tone data, most experienced audiologists will be able to ascertain inconsistent responses for speech testing that can lead to the diagnosis of a functional hearing loss.

Another test that can be done to determine whether a functional hearing loss is present is the Stenger Test. The Stenger Test can be done using either pure tone or speech stimuli. This test is used to identify the presence of a functional hearing loss when an asymmetrical hearing loss of at least 20 dB HL exists (Katz, 2002). The theory behind the Stenger is that when both ears are stimulated simultaneously the auditory stimulus will lateralize to the better ear. The stimulus is presented to the better ear at 10 dB HL above the threshold, and the stimulus is presented at 10 dB HL below that volunteered threshold in the poorer ear. If the stimulus is louder in the poorer ear, then the individual will not report hearing the tone or speech stimulus. This is referred to as a *Positive Stenger* and suggests the presence of a functional hearing loss.

Whenever possible the audiologist should try to resolve the functional component of the hearing loss to obtain reliable and valid test results. If the functional component of the hearing loss cannot be resolved, then the patient and family should be referred for further professional services such as psychological counseling, with audiologic retesting following any intervention.

SPEECH AUDIOMETRY

Speech audiometry is used to diagnose the type and degree of hearing loss, determine the site of lesion in the auditory system, and assess possible candidacy for audiologic rehabilitation such as hearing aids. Speech audiometry is used to support the reliability of other audiologic tests. Speech audiometry may be conducted as threshold or suprathreshold measurements. The overall goal of the testing is to obtain information about speech understanding in a variety of listening conditions (e.g., quiet and noise). Routine speech audiometric testing will be discussed in this section. More specialized speech testing will be addressed in other sections of this textbook.

Speech Recognition Threshold/Speech Reception Threshold

The speech recognition threshold/speech reception threshold (SRT) is defined as the lowest intensity level at which 50% of spondee stimuli are repeated correctly. According to Martin and Dowdy (1986), the SRT is achieved when three correct responses have been obtained at a given hearing level. Spondee words are two-syllable words with equal stress on each syllable. Spondees are selected from the CID (Central Institute for the Deaf) W-1 word lists, which are comprised of 36 spondees (Martin & Weller, 1975). For children or adults who may not be able to verbally respond, the SRT testing can be accomplished using a spondee picture board or spondee objects (e.g., toothbrush, airplane, baseball). In cases of severe hearing loss or speech-language deficits, a selected spondee word list can be used. A select spondee list of 6 to 8 words, rather than the entire 36-spondee list, can be presented to obtain the threshold. When a selected list of spondee words is used, the SRT may be lower or better because the patient is selecting the response from a closed set rather than an open set of spondees, the former being an easier task.

The use of a selected list should be noted on the audiogram. The SRT serves as a reliability check on the pure tone thresholds obtained in the speech frequencies of 500 Hz, 1000 Hz, and 2000 Hz. It also provides a reference level for suprathreshold speech measurements. When the pure tone and speech results are reliable, the thresholds will be within ± 5 dB HL. When there is a discrepancy between these thresholds, the audiologist must ascertain the possible reason(s) for the inconsistencies. The discrepancies may be related to poor instructions, lack of understanding the instructions, functional hearing loss, or lack of equipment calibration. The astute clinician should be able to predict the SRT based on the PTA to ascertain the reliability and validity of the patient's responses.

Speech Detection Threshold/Speech Awareness Threshold

The speech detection threshold (SDT), also called the speech awareness threshold (SAT), is obtained for patients who cannot complete SRT testing, such young children and individuals with speech-language-hearing disorders or cognitive impairment. In such cases, the SDT/SAT is preferable to the SRT. The SDT/SAT is defined as the lowest intensity level at which an individual can detect the presence of speech 50% of the time. The patient does not need to identify the speech stimuli but only be aware that speech is present. In most cases the SDT/SAT will be lower or better than the pure tone thresholds by approximately 10–15 dB HL. The most common speech stimuli used to obtain the SDT/SAT are continuous discourse and cold running speech.

Word Recognition Score

Word recognition performance estimates the ability of patients to understand words presented at suprathreshold hearing levels, typically 40 dB HL above the SRT (re: SRT) (Katz, 2002). The main purpose of word recognition testing is to evaluate speech understanding when words are presented at a loud intensity level in a variety of listening conditions. The most commonly used monosyllabic stimuli are the Northwestern University (NU#6) and the Central Institute for the Deaf (CID W-22) phonetically balanced (PB) word lists. Phonetically balanced word lists contain speech sounds that occur with the same frequency as in conversational speech (Stach, 1999). Typically, word recognition testing is conducted initially at 40 dB SL above the SRT (i.e., re: SRT) or at the patient's most comfortable listening level (MCL) for speech. However, these levels may not represent the patient's maximum word recognition score. The maximum word recognition score may be obtained by testing at several intensity levels, referred to as a Phonetically Balanced Performance Intensity (PB-PI) function. At some intensity level on the PB-PI function, a point will be reached at which the patient's maximum word recognition score is achieved and increasing the intensity level of the speech stimuli will not yield a better score. This is referred to as the PB-PI plateau. Typically, the testing is initiated at 40 dB SL re: SRT and proceeds in increments of 10 dB SL until the maximum power output of the audiometer for speech is attained. The PB-PI function has several diagnostic and rehabilitation applications. This function can help to determine the site of lesion in the auditory system. In cases of conductive, cochlear, or mixed hearing losses, as intensity increases the PB score also increases until an intensity level is reached at which the word recognition score plateaus. In cases of retrocochlear hearing loss, as intensity level is increased an individual's PB score will decrease. This phenomenon, known as PB-PI rollover, is a classic sign of retrocochlear involvement, such as an VIII nerve tumor, and requires further neuro-otologic assessment.

For word recognition testing, if a 25-word list is used, then each correct word receives a score of 4%. If a 50-word list is used, then each correct word receives a score of 2%. The maximum score that can be attained is 100%, with a minimum score of 0%. The higher the score, the better the individual's word recognition ability (see Table 1.3). Individuals with good word recognition scores are candidates for audiologic rehabilitation.

Word recognition testing can be done using a variety of test stimuli including nonsense syllables, monosyllabic words, and sentences. The most difficult speech materials for patients with hearing loss are nonsense syllables, followed by monosyllabic words as the second most difficult, with sentences being the easiest task. The type of speech material selected depends on how the test results will be used. For example, in determining site of lesion, it is critical to obtain a PB-PI function for monosyllabic words to assess whether rollover is present. If the audiologist would like to obtain information related to auditory processing ability, it is better to use degraded tests such as the Synthetic Sentence Identification (SSI), Staggered Spondaic Word (SSW), Hearing in Noise Test (HINT), Quick Speech in Noise Test (Quick SIN), or Speech Perception In Noise (SPIN). The auditory processing test selected will be based on the population under investigation, the amount of time allotted to conduct the test, and the audiologist's expertise in administering and interpreting the test data. More important, the speech test selected is based on how the test results will be used for diagnostic and rehabilitation purposes.

Loudness Level

Most comfortable listening level for speech. In determining if a patient might be eligible for amplification, it is recommended that the most comfortable listening (MCL) level for speech be established. The MCL is defined as the hearing intensity level an individual reports to be the most comfortable for listening to speech for an extended period of time (Katz, 2002). This suprathreshold measurement is typically obtained using running speech stimuli. For normal hearing adults, the MCL is usually around 40–55 dB HL above the SRT. For individuals with hearing loss, the MCL will be affected by the degree and type of hearing loss. For example, a reduced or low MCL may suggest physiological recruitment due to cochlear or retrocochlear involvement. The MCL is a valuable measurement that can be used in the fitting of hearing aids, assistive listening devices, and

TABLE 1.3 Interpretation of Word Recognition Score in Percent (%) Correct

% Correct Score	Interpretation
96–100%	Excellent
88–94%	Very good
80–86%	Good
70–78%	Fair
50–68%	Poor
< 50%	Very Poor

Adapted from Stach, B. (1999). *Clinical audiology: An introduction.* San Diego: Singular.

Speech Audiometry

cochlear implants. An MCL also can be obtained for pure tone stimuli at different frequencies. It is cautioned that these measurements are time-consuming and typically are not done on a routine basis. However, specific MCL thresholds provide valuable information for hearing aid evaluations and mapping for cochlear implantation.

Loudness discomfort level/uncomfortable listening level for speech. Valuable information can be attained for hearing aid fittings and cochlear implantation mapping by establishing a patient's loudness discomfort level (LDL) or uncomfortable listening level (UCL). The LDL/UCL is defined as the loudest level at which an individual can tolerate sound without experiencing physiologic pain (Katz, 2002). This suprathreshold measurement is obtained using running speech stimuli. Most individuals with normal hearing and conductive hearing loss can tolerate as much as 100–105 dB HL of sound without reaching a level of discomfort. For individuals with cochlear hearing loss, the LDL/UCL may be reduced below 90 dB HL, which may be indicative of physiological recruitment (Katz, 2002). As is the case with MCL, the audiologist can establish LDL/UCL measurements for pure tone stimuli. The difference between the patient's LDL/UCL for speech and the SRT provides information on the dynamic range of hearing. The wider the dynamic range, the easier it is to fit amplification for the patient. For example, if the LDL/UCL is 100 dB HL and the SRT is 40 dB HL, then the dynamic range is 60 dB HL. If there is a reduced dynamic range, then compression may be necessary when recommending hearing aids.

Masking for Speech Audiometry

Masking for speech is required when there is a possibility of the nontest ear participating in the speech testing due to cross-hearing. The interaural attenuation value for speech is 50 dB HL when using supra-aural earphones. The interaural attenuation value for speech is 70 dB HL when using insert earphones. When conducting suprathreshold speech audiometry, the need for masking the nontest ear is determined by evaluating the presentation level minus the interaural attenuation and determining whether the amount of sound crossing over can be heard by the best bone conduction threshold of the nontest ear. If the answer is yes, then masking is necessary.

According to Martin and Clark (2005) the formula used to determine the initial masking level for speech masking is as follows:

PL (presentation level) – IA (interaural attenuation) > the best bone conduction thresholds in the nontest ear

For speech audiometry, it is not necessary to use the plateau method as is done for pure tone testing. It is only necessary to present one level of noise to the nontest ear at each designated testing level. The type of noise used is speech spectrum, as it provides more energy in the low frequencies mimicking the speech spectrum. The following decisions need to be made when determining the need to mask for speech testing (Martin & Clarke, 2005). The following are questions to answer to determine the masking level:

1. What is the presentation level for the speech stimuli in the test ear?

2. Will cross-hearing occur via the best bone conduction threshold in the nontest ear at the designated presentation level? If yes, what amount of sound is crossing over via bone conduction to the nontest ear?

3. How much does the best bone conduction threshold need to be shifted in order for cross-hearing not to occur in the nontest ear?

4. How much does the air conduction threshold need to be shifted in order to shift the bone conduction threshold so that cross-hearing is eliminated for speech testing?

5. What is the effective masking level at each speech presentation level for the nontest ear?

Students and novice clinicians tend to understand masking principles for speech audiometry more easily than masking concepts for pure tone audiometry. Once students grasp the concepts of masking for pure tones, then it is easy to conceptualize masking for speech audiometry.

Issues in Speech Audiometry

There are several issues that must be considered when conducting speech audiometry testing. Some factors include recorded versus live voice testing, number of test stimuli to present, presentation level, response mode, use of a carrier phrase, and type of test condition. Each factor will be addressed briefly. For more information on this topic, refer to the Recommended Readings provided at the end of this part.

Test environment. The test environment in which speech audiometry is conducted should meet the current ANSI standards for acceptable levels of ambient noise (1999). The speech mode of the audiometer also should meet the current ANSI (1996) specification for audiometers.

Presentation of full-list versus half-list speech stimuli. There is controversy among audiologists as to whether a 25-word or a 50-word list should be presented for word recognition testing. The number of words presented has a direct relationship to the reliability of the test scores. Thornton and Raffin (1978) presented a critical difference model to help determine whether there is a significant difference in word recognition scores depending on the number of words presented. They stated that the half-list of 25 words can be as reliable as the full 50-word list. Thorton and Raffin (1978) also noted that, the smaller the number of test items, the larger the test-retest difference score needed to establish confidence limits. The authors put forth lower and upper limits of the 95% critical differences for percentage scores as a function of test and sample size. If the actual score obtained on the second test as compared to the first test is outside the range, then the two scores are considered to be significantly different. For example, when the word recognition score is 80%, there is a 95% probability that the score on another form of the test would fall between 64% and 92% on a 50-item test and between 56% and 96% on a 25-item list. When the score on the second test is outside the predicted range, the scores can be considered significantly different and therefore would not contribute to the diagnostic information about the hearing loss. In most clinics, due to time constraints, most audiologists use 25 words for routine word recognition testing, which may compromise the test results.

Presentation level of speech stimuli. Martin, Champlin, and Chambers (1998) surveyed audiologists regarding their clinical practices and found that the majority use a variety of methods to select the presentation level in assessing suprathreshold word recognition ability. In their study, 75% of audiologists reported presenting the speech stimuli at 40 dB SL re: SRT. Twenty percent of audiologists reported using the MCL for word recognition testing, whereas other audiologists reported conducting speech recognition testing at several intensity levels. The major problem with presenting words at one fixed level is that the patient's maximum word recognition score known as PB Max may not be obtained. It may be necessary in such cases to conduct word recognition testing at several presentation levels, especially if the initial score is either poor or one that may not be expected based on pure tone results. Word recognition testing should be conducted at a minimum of two levels between 50 dB HL and 90 dB HL. Testing at several intensity levels will help the audiologist determine the site of lesion in the auditory mechanism and also provide information on the patient's maximum word/speech recognition score. Such information is helpful for fitting amplification devices.

Recorded versus monitored live-voice testing. One issue in contention in clinical practice is whether speech stimuli should be presented via monitored live voice or recorded. Although there are advantages of using monitored live-voice testing, including saving time, the test results may be altered by the audiologist's accent or pronunciation. Due to time constraints, most audiologists use 25-word lists presented via monitored live voice. This issue has several ramifications for a patient's performance and the outcome of the word recognition test results. The use of monitored live-voice testing may compromise the reliability and validity of the test results because the speech of the audiologist may vary when testing the same patient or different patients. However, there are some patients for whom it is necessary to complete the testing in a rapid manner (e.g., children or elderly with cognitive impairment). For the majority of patients, it is best to present speech using recorded materials. The use of recorded materials allows for comparison of test scores for different test sessions as well as across clinics (Katz, 2002).

Use of carrier phrase. For word recognition testing, a carrier phrase such as "say the word" is used preceding the presence of the monosyllabic word. The carrier phrase is used to calibrate the speech signal so that the proper intensity is achieved. If a carrier phrase is not used, then what are the ramifications on word recognition testing? Katz (2002) reported that when a carrier phrase is not used for suprathreshold word recognition, the scores tend to be poorer. It is best to be conservative and use a carrier phrase for word recognition so that the test results are not compromised during live-voice testing. The carrier phrase is always included in the recorded speech materials for standardization purposes.

Test condition.   The most common method of assessing speech recognition ability is at a suprathreshold level in quiet. It is useful for audiologists to assess speech understanding in noise, as this is more representative of how an individual with hearing loss will communicate in the noisy listening situations that are typical of daily communication environments. One of the major problems with conducting speech-in-noise measurements is that the interpretation of the results is controversial. At present, there are no norms to interpret speech-in-noise results. If the results are poor, then it may be surmised that the individual may be experiencing hearing problems in noise. In addition, for speech-in-noise assessment, there is not a standard message-to-competition ratio that is used (e.g., 0 S/N, +10 S/N, –10 S/N). It is recommended that testing be done at several message-to-competition ratios including a + signal-to-noise ratio, at which the speech signal is louder than the competing noise; a zero (0) signal-to-noise ratio, at which the speech and noise are presented at the same intensity level; and a – signal-to-noise ratio, at which the competing noise is presented at a louder level than the speech signal.

Response mode.   The most common response mode for speech testing from the patient is a verbal response. For those individuals who may not be able to respond verbally, it may be necessary either to obtain a written response or to use pointing to a picture as the response task. One issue to consider is that an open response paradigm is subject to the audiologist's interpretation of a correct verbal response, whereas a picture-point or written response is easier to interpret. The type of response mode can have a significant effect on the speech recognition score. In a closed response set, the patient will be able to select the stimulus from a group of, typically, four or six alternatives. In contrast, the open-set response consists of no specific target stimulus. In the latter condition, the patient can select any word from a lexicon of thousands of possible alternatives, which makes answering a more difficult task (Stach, 1999).

Soundfield Speech Audiometry

Speech stimuli can be presented in the soundfield, which involves presenting acoustic stimuli through loudspeaker(s) in a calibrated test environment. Typically, the speech stimuli are presented through speakers positioned at a 0-, 40-, or 60-degree azimuth (Katz, 2002). The major problem with soundfield testing is that it is not certain which ear is responding because the ears are not isolated. Consequently, both ears may be responding in a symmetrical hearing loss; in cases of asymmetrical hearing loss, it is probably the better ear responding. Soundfield testing is often done as part of a hearing aid evaluation in order to assess a patient's ability to understand speech in a variety of listening situations such as quiet or in the presence of competing noise at various signal-to-noise ratios.

Testing Culturally and Linguistically Diverse Patients

Due to the increase in the number of individuals in the United States who are non-English speakers, it is necessary for audiologists to try to obtain critical information related to communication abilities via speech audiometry. If the audiologist is not bilingual, then it may be necessary to use an interpreter or be assisted by a family member who is bilingual. Some speech materials are available in Spanish, Yiddish, and Russian. It is critical that the profession of audiology develop more culturally sensitive materials in order to accommodate the speech and language needs of an increasingly diverse population in the United States and throughout the world. Word recognition testing should be done in the patient's primary language in order to ascertain reliable and valid assessment of communication difficulties.

Recording Speech Audiometry Results on the Audiogram

The results of the speech data are recorded in the designated spaces on the audiogram. For the ASHA audiogram (2003), there is a specific section for recording the SRT or SAT/SDT. There is a separate section on the audiogram to record word recognition test results, and it includes information for recording the presentation level and the masking level for each ear. There are also checkboxes for the type of speech material used as well as the method of delivery of the speech materials. MCL and LDL/UCL for speech can also be recorded in this section of the audiogram. Soundfield test results also are recorded when assessed including presentation level and test condition. As with pure tone audiometry, any modifications to speech audiometric testing needs to be documented in the comment section of the audiogram.

Most audiologists will use the results of the word recognition testing to try to predict the communication problems encounters on a daily basis. There is a great deal of variability across individuals related to their performance on speech measures as a function of hearing loss. Some of these factors include cognitive and personality variables. In terms of how speech recognition scores correlate with daily communication abilities, most audiologists will base their predictions of communication problems on clinical experience. Speech audiometric results are critical in determining candidacy for amplification and other forms of audiologic rehabilitation intervention.

OBJECTIVE ASSESSMENT OF THE AUDITORY SYSTEM

There are several objective tests that can be done to assess the status of the auditory system. These tests can provide a myriad of information especially for difficult-to-test populations for whom routine audiometric testing may yield inconsistent test results. The tests that will be described in this section include immittance testing and auditory evoked potentials. Immittance testing is typically a part of a routine audiologic evaluation for most children and adults. OAEs are usually done for screening purposes, when a functional or ototoxic hearing loss is suspected. Auditory-evoked potentials are used to assess the neurological integrity of the auditory system from the VIII nerve to the auditory cortex. Early auditory brainstem responses (ABR) can be used to estimate hearing threshold levels, later auditory potentials provide information about cognitive functioning. A general overview of these tests is provided. For more detailed information, refer to the References and Recommended Reading lists in this textbook.

Acoustic Immittance Battery

One of the most valuable objective tools used to assess middle-ear function is the acoustic immittance battery. It is highly recommended that the immittance battery be a routine component of the basic audiologic assessment. The battery consists of tympanometry, acoustic static compliance, acoustic reflex thresholds, and acoustic reflex decay. The results provide information about whether there is medical pathology in the middle-ear system and also can provide additional information on the location of the site of lesion in the auditory system (i.e., cochlear vs. retrocochlear). The acoustic reflex data from the immittance battery can be used to estimate hearing thresholds levels with good predictability when compared to pure tone thresholds. Each component of the acoustic immittance battery will be reviewed briefly.

Tympanometry. Tympanometry is an objective assessment of the status of the middle ear. It measures the immittance characteristics of the middle-ear system as a function of changes in air pressure in the external auditory canal. Tympanometry is a dynamic measurement of eardrum mobility as air pressure is varied from +200 daPa to –200 daPa in the ear canal. When there is positive air pressure, the tympanic membrane moves inward toward the middle-ear cavity, resulting in resistance in the middle-ear system and a great deal of reflection of sound. In a normal ear, when air pressure varies from +200 daPa to 0 daPa, there is a reduction in the amount of resistance, and more sound enters into the middle ear system. In the case of a normal middle-ear system, equal air pressure will be near 0 daPa, which is the point of maximum compliance. As air pressure varies from 0 daPa to –200 daPa, there is an increase in resistance, and sound is reflected from the eardrum.

Pathology in the external or middle ear will change the stiffness, mass, and/or resistance of the middle-ear system. The point of maximum compliance will result in equal amount of air pressure on both sides of the eardrum, which usually occurs between +100 and –100 daPa in adults and +150 and –150 daPa in children (Jerger, 1970). The tympanogram is a graphic display of tympanometry data. The tympanometric pattern depicting middle-ear pressure and eardrum mobility will help determine the pathology in the middle-ear system. Jerger (1970) put forth the following tympanogram patterns to help identify the pathology in the middle-ear system (see Figure 1.3).

Objective Assessment of the Auditory System

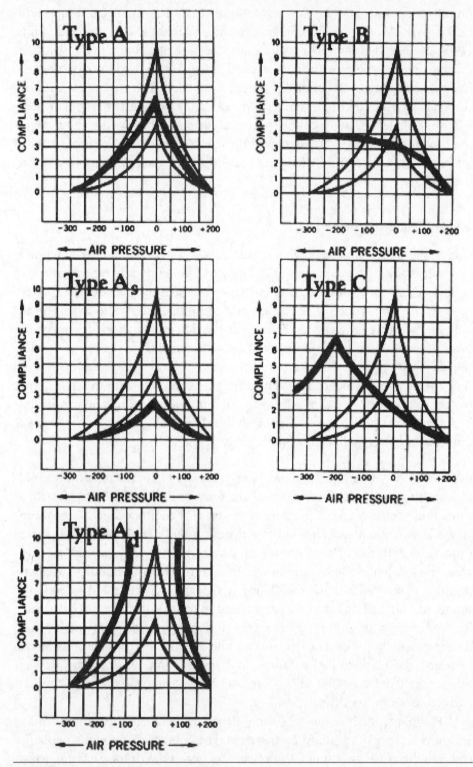

FIGURE 1.3 Tympanogram Patterns

Reprinted with permission from Jerger, J. (1970). Clinical experience with impedance audiometry. *Archives of Otolaryngology, 92,* 311–324. Copyright © 1970 American Medical Association. All rights reserved.

PART 1 Audiometric Testing Principles and Audiogram Interpretation

TYPE A

- Normal middle-ear pressure with normal tympanic membrane mobility
- No middle-ear pathology
- Normal hearing or sensorineural hearing loss

TYPE A$_S$

- Normal middle-ear pressure with reduced (i.e., shallow) tympanic membrane mobility
- Middle-ear system with mass and high resistance
- Common in otosclerosis, cholesteatoma, tympanosclerosis, and ossicular fixation

TYPE A$_D$

- Normal middle-ear pressure with excessive tympanic membrane mobility
- Highly compliant middle-ear system with little resistance
- Common in ossicular discontinuity; flaccid tympanic membrane or tympanic membrane perforation

TYPE C

- Negative middle-ear pressure with normal tympanic membrane mobility
- Common in Eustachian tube dysfunction and early or resolving otitis media

TYPE B

- No point of maximum compliance with extremely reduced tympanic membrane mobility (e.g., flat)
- Common in perforated tympanic membrane, impacted cerumen, advanced otitis media, or a benign cholesteatoma

Static acoustic compliance. Static acoustic compliance measures the volume of the middle-ear system in cubic centimeters (cc) or milliliters (ml). Static acoustic compliance is used to determine the degree of stiffness of the tympanic membrane and the ossicular chain in the middle ear. If there is a pathology in the middle-ear system, then the static compliance value will be affected. Some pathologies, such as a perforated eardrum or ossicular discontinuity, will cause the volume in the middle ear to be larger, whereas other pathologies, such as a tumor or fluid, will cause the volume to be reduced due to mass in the middle ear. Normal static compliance values for children age 3 to 10 years range from 0.25 ml to .05 ml. The range is 0.30 ml–1.70 ml for patients 18 years of age and older. Static compliance values need to be interpreted as part of the immittance battery in order to have clinical significance. These values should not be used for making clinical decisions in isolation but interpreted as part of the immit-

Objective Assessment of the Auditory System

tance test battery to determine the physiological status of the middle-ear system (Jerger, 1970).

Acoustic reflex thresholds.   Acoustic reflex thresholds are a bilateral contraction of the tensor tympani and stapedius muscles of the middle ear in response to high levels of acoustic stimulation that typically exceed 90 dB SPL (i.e., sound pressure level). They can be measured in the ear contralateral to stimulation (i.e., contralateral acoustic reflexes) or the ear ipsilateral (i.e., ipsilateral acoustic reflex) to stimulation with a probe tone of 226 Hz. Other frequencies such as 660 Hz are available in commercial units. The acoustic reflex threshold is the lowest stimulus intensity at which a change in immittance can be identified by visually monitoring the needle deflection on the immittance equipment. Contralateral acoustic reflexes are measured bilaterally at 500 Hz, 1000 Hz, 2000 Hz, and 4000 Hz, whereas ipsilateral acoustic reflexes are measured at 500 Hz, 1000 Hz, and 2000 Hz. Typically, in cases of conductive or mixed hearing loss, the acoustic reflex thresholds may be elevated or absent. In cases of sensorineural hearing loss that is cochlear in nature, the acoustic reflex thresholds may be present at reduced levels depending on the degree of hearing loss. In cases of severe-to-profound hearing loss, the acoustic reflex thresholds typically cannot be measured due to the severity of the hearing loss. In general, when hearing loss exceeds 70 dB HL, it is difficult to obtain reflexes because the equipment cannot produce sufficient sound intensity to elicit them. The level at which the acoustic reflexes are present can provide information to predict hearing loss. In addition, the acoustic reflex thresholds will provide valuable information about the site of lesion in the auditory system. They are very sensitive in assessing whether there is VII or VIII nerve involvement, such as a tumor.

Relationship between hearing loss and acoustic reflex thresholds.   The following are typical patterns of acoustic reflex thresholds based on the type and degree of hearing loss:

> *Conductive hearing loss*—In conductive hearing loss, the acoustic reflex thresholds may not be elicited for contralateral and ipsilateral stimulation due to the presence of middle-ear pathology. In conductive hearing loss, the acoustic reflexes will typically be absent in the probe ear for one of two reasons. The first reason is that the pathology in the middle-ear system prohibits the contraction of the reflex. The second reason is that the change in the muscle contraction is not large enough to produce a change in immittance recorded at the probe tip. In conductive hearing loss in which the acoustic reflexes are elicited, they may be present at elevated levels in the ear with the conductive pathology.

> *Sensorineural-cochlear hearing loss*—The acoustic reflex thresholds can be measured in cases of sensorineural hearing loss up to 45 dB HL. As the hearing loss increases, acoustic reflexes may be present at reduced sensation levels suggesting cochlear involvement. When cochlear hearing loss exceeds 70 dB HL, the acoustic reflex usually will not be measurable.

Sensorineural-retrocochlear hearing loss—There are several patterns that can emerge in cases of retrocochlear involvement depending on whether a hearing loss is present. When contralateral acoustic reflexes are present, they may be elicited at elevated sensation levels relative to the hearing loss. Another common pattern in retrocochlear hearing loss is that the expected acoustic reflexes are not present in normal hearing or a mild hearing loss.

Acoustic reflex decay.   When contralateral acoustic reflexes are elicited, an additional test referred to as acoustic reflex decay can be done. Acoustic reflex decay is measured by presenting a continuous tone for 10 seconds at 10 dB SL above the contralateral acoustic reflex threshold at 500 Hz and 1000 Hz. Acoustic reflex decay is not measured at 2000 Hz or 4000 Hz because decay can be present in normal ears. At these frequencies in cases of conductive, mixed, and cochlear hearing loss, the reflexes will be able to sustain a contraction for a duration of 10 seconds. In retrocochlear involvement, the acoustic reflex cannot be maintained for the 10 second duration, and acoustic reflex decay will be present, usually during the first 5 seconds of stimulation (Katz, 2002). Acoustic reflex decay is defined as a decrease in amplitude of 50% or greater from the initial onset. When present, it is reported as positive acoustic reflex decay. The immittance battery provides a broad range of information about the middle ear and the acoustic reflex arch that is critical for diagnosis of the site of lesion of the hearing loss.

Otoacoustic Emissions

An objective assessment that is gaining in popularity is the otoacoustic emissions (OAEs) described by Kemp (1978). OAEs are useful for determining whether a hearing loss is cochlear in origin. According to Kemp (1978), OAEs are generated from the outer hair cells of the cochlea. OAEs are not a measurement of hearing sensitivity; rather, they provide information about the status of the outer hair cells in cochlea. There are two categories of OAEs: spontaneous emissions and evoked emissions. Spontaneous emissions do not require a stimulus to evoke them because they are present naturally in the cochlea. The second type, known as evoked emissions, requires an external stimulus to elicit the cochlear response. OAEs will be present in normal hearing and where a cochlear hearing loss does not exceed 30–40 dB HL (Kemp, 1978). Cochlear emissions will not be present in cases of conductive pathology because the emissions cannot be picked up by the microphone in the external auditory canal due to the presence of outer- and/or middle-ear pathology.

Two types of evoked OAEs are transient evoked otoacoustic emissions (TEOAEs) and distortion product otoacoustic emissions (DPOAEs). DPOAEs allow the audiologist to assess different frequency regions in the auditory system from 1000 Hz to 8000 Hz for hearing loss up to about 45–55 dB HL. TEOAEs are typically not seen in individuals with a hearing loss greater than 30–35 dB HL (i.e., mild) (Kemp, 1978).

Three factors that must be present in order to obtain reliable and valid OAEs include (1) a relaxed patient, to avoid a high rejection rate due to patient artifact; (2) low background noise, so as not to interfere with test stimuli; and (3) a well-fitted probe, to ensure a good seal so that the microphone can pick up the cochlear emissions in the ear canal. OAEs are typically used as a screening tool for neonates in universal hearing screening programs. They also have utility in cases of functional hearing loss and are useful in monitoring the ototoxic effects on the outer hair cells in the cochlea. OAEs are reliable, quick, consistent, and cost-effective. Therefore, they are a good tool for audiologic assessment of the status of the outer hair cells of the cochlea.

Auditory Brainstem Response

The auditory brainstem response (ABR) is an objective assessment of the neurological integrity of the cochlea and the auditory brainstem (Hall, 2007). The ABR provides information about the neurological integrity from VIII nerve to the brainstem. In addition, it is used to estimate auditory thresholds for patients (e.g., pediatric, mentally challenged, elderly with cognitive impairment) who are unable to provide voluntary thresholds. The ABR consists of five waveforms that occur within the first 7 to 10 ms of acoustic stimulation. The acoustic stimuli used to elicit the ABR are either clicks or tone bursts/tone pips (Hall, 2007). In order to record the ABR, an array of electrodes are placed on the head and ears. For neurological purposes, the latencies at which the waves are present provide information about the integrity of the auditory system. Waves I and II are thought to be generated by the VIII nerve ipsilateral to stimulation. The remaining waves are thought to be generated by ipsilateral, contralateral, and bilateral structures in the auditory brainstem. The absolute latency is defined as the time of occurrence of an evoked potential, that is, as the time between the presentation of a stimulus and the peak of the potential. The absolute latency at which waves I, II, III, IV, and V are present is calculated. Typically, the absolute latency of wave I is 1.0 msec; wave II, 2.0 msec; wave III, 3.0 msec; wave IV, 4.0 msec; and wave V, 5.0 msec (Hall, 2007). In addition to the absolute latency, the relative interpeak latency between waves I to III, I to V, and III to V is calculated. An ABR is considered to be abnormal when one or more of the following conditions are present: Relative interpeak intervals are prolonged especially for waves I-V, the morphology of wave V is significantly different between ears, and/or wave V is prolonged or absent at high-click-rate stimulation. Due to limitations in using solely the absolute latency of wave V, such as effects of sensorineural hearing loss, wide distribution of wave V latencies across normal individuals, and different variables that affect wave V such as body temperature and head size, it is preferred to use the interaural comparisons of wave V latency to determine whether an VIII nerve tumor is present (Hall, 2007).

In addition to wave latencies, the amplitudes of waves I, III, and V are analyzed to determine whether they are present at reduced amplitude measurements. The absolute amplitude is measured peak-to-peak of the wave. The relative amplitude is defined as the magnitude of the potential relative to the magnitude of another potential. An analysis of the morphology of the waveform is critical in assessing the neurological integrity of the auditory system. Oftentimes in cases of retrocochlear involvement, the morphology of the waveform is compromised due to the pathology in the auditory system.

A second use of the ABR is to estimate hearing thresholds in patients for whom it is difficult to obtain accurate behavioral measurements. In such instances the presence of wave V is used to estimate the hearing threshold levels by evaluating the lowest intensity level at which wave V is present. A latency-intensity function that depicts the presence of wave V as a function of intensity is generated. The threshold for wave V using toneburst stimuli has been estimated to be within 15 dB HL of the patient's behavioral threshold for frequencies of 1000 Hz to 4000 Hz. The lowest intensity level at which wave V is present is considered to be an estimation of a behavioral hearing threshold level (Hall, 2007).

ABR results provide audiologists with extensive information to determine type and degree of hearing loss. Objective information from the ABR is critical in the diagnosis of hearing loss in some young children and difficult-to-test populations. The ABR is a very powerful electrophysiological assessment tool. The later auditory potentials, such as the Middle Latency Response (MLR), typically occur between 10 and 50 msec, and the late evoked potential such as P_{300} occurs around 300 msec after the stimulus onset (Hall, 2007). These electrophysiological auditory assessments can provide information about levels higher in the brainstem and auditory cortex. The later auditory potentials are being used more frequently as part of the audiologist's test battery, especially as related to speech perception abilities (e.g., P_{300}).

One new method of detecting VIII tumors, especially those that are small, is the stacked ABR. It is beyond the scope of this introductory textbook to address the value of the stacked ABR in neuro-otology. For further information on this technique, refer to Hall (2007).

Relationship between site of lesion and ABR results.   The following summarizes the effect of each type of hearing loss on ABR results.

> *Conductive hearing loss*—Wave I is delayed due to conductive hearing loss. Interpeak intervals are within normal limits.
>
> *Sensorineural hearing loss*—Wave I is delayed due to the hearing loss. Interpeak latencies are within normal limits, and interpeak latency of waves I–V may be shortened due to the delay of wave I.
>
> *Retrocochlear hearing loss*—Wave I is usually within normal latency period, whereas waves III and V may be delayed. Interpeak latencies also may be delayed for I–III, I–V, and III–V.

RECORDING AUDIOLOGICAL DATA

The audiogram should include the following information: unmasked and masked pure tone air and bone conduction thresholds (when appropriate, the level of masking noise should be included), speech audiometric results, and the level of speech-masking noise when used. Tympanogram, acoustic reflex thresholds, and acoustic reflex decay results should be recorded when done. There should also be a comments section to record information about the patient's responses or any other valuable information related to the test session. There should be a section on the audiogram that relates to the reliability of the patient's responses. Any inconsistencies in the patient's behavior and/or test results should be documented.

It is very beneficial for students to record all test data on one audiogram. For example, results from the immittance battery should be recorded on the same audiogram as the pure tone and speech data. From a pedagogical perspective, students can interpret each test independently and as part of the whole battery.

In summary, the combination of objective and behavioral auditory assessments are powerful diagnostic tools. The audiologist has a selection of numerous behavioral and objective assessments to assist in the determination of type and degree of hearing loss. It is critical that students integrate the information provided by each test to gain a complete picture of the auditory system and the possible etiology of the hearing loss. An accurate diagnosis of the hearing loss is critical in order to make the appropriate audiologic rehabilitation decision to improve a patient's communication abilities.

The remainder of this part will provide the student with case history information and behavioral and/or objective auditory assessments to use to diagnose the hearing loss for each case presented. Students are challenged to answer questions based on the audiologic information. In addition, the Clinical Enrichment Projects offer students opportunities to expand their theoretical and clinical knowledge on a variety of topics in audiology related to the case studies presented.

Audiogram Interpretation Exercises

Mr. J., a 40-year-old male, was seen for a routine audiologic evaluation. He reported being in excellent physical health. Mr. J. stated that he has been experiencing a continuous high-pitched ringing sound in both ears that began about one month ago. He said that over the last year it appears that his hearing has been declining. He experiences difficulty hearing especially when listening to music. He has been a musician playing the clarinet in a local orchestra for the last 10 years. He has never used hearing protection. Mr. J. stated that after practice or a performance he cannot hear for about a day and experiences tinnitus in both ears. Mr. J.'s father had a hearing loss and wore hearing aids. There is no other significant medical, audiologic, or otologic history. (See Figure 1.4.)

1. Describe the hearing sensitivity in each ear.

2. Calculate the three-frequency pure tone average in each ear.

3. Are the SRTs in good agreement with the PTAs bilaterally? Why?

4. What was the presentation level of the NU#6 word lists in each ear? How would you describe the word recognition results in each ear with regard to communication abilities?

5. Describe the results of the immittance battery for each ear.

6. What audiologic recommendations do you have for this patient?

NAME: Patient 1   AGE/DATE OF BIRTH: 40 y/o

REFERRED BY: _____   MEDICAL RECORD #: _____

TEST INTERVAL: _____   DATE OF TEST: _____

PURE TONE AUDIOMETRY (RE: ANSI 1996)

KEY:

	LEFT	Stimulus	RIGHT	
X		AIR		O
□		AIR - MASK		Δ
>		BONE		<
↘		BONE - MASK		[
		NO RESPONSE		↓
L		AIDED SOUND FIELD		R
		SOUND FIELD = S		

TEST TYPE
STANDARD OAE
PLAY
COR/VRA
BOA

TRANSDUCER
INSERT
CIRCUMAURAL
SOUND FIELD

RELIABILITY
EXCELLENT
GOOD
FAIR
POOR

BOOTH
#1
#2 (PEDS)
#3
#4 COCH IMPLANT

TYMPANOMETRY (226 Hz)

EAR	LEFT	RIGHT
STATIC ADMITTANCE (mm H₂O)		
TYMP PEAK PRESSURE (DaPa)		
TYMP WIDTH (DaPa)		
EAR CANAL VOLUME cm³	.69	.74

LEFT   RIGHT   Admittance

Pressure   Pressure

CONTRA	.5k Hz	1k Hz	2k Hz	4k Hz	IPSI	.5k Hz	1k Hz	2k Hz	4k Hz
Right (AD) (phone ear)	85	85	90	90	AD (probe ear)	85	85	90	
Left (AS) (phone ear)	85	85	90	90	AS (probe ear)	80	85	90	

MIDDLE EAR ANALYZER _____

SPEECH AUDIOMETRY

	PTA	SRT/SAT	Speech Recognition	Speech Recognition	MCL	UCL
RIGHT (AD)	10		50 dBHL			
Masking		100 %		%		
LEFT (AS)	10		50 dBHL			
Masking		100%		%		

MLV □	CD/tape ☒	W-22 □	WIPI □	PBK □	SPECIAL: NU #6	SPECIAL:
SOUND FIELD			%		%	
RIGHT AIDED			%		%	
LEFT AIDED			%		%	
BINAURAL			%		%	

OTOACOUSTIC EMISSIONS (OAEs)

EMISSION TYPE USED	TEST TYPE PERFORMED
Transient	OAE Complete
Distortion Product	OAE Screening
OAE results:	
Right Ear	
Left Ear	

OAE UNIT _____

HEARING AID INFORMATION

RIGHT AID: _____

LEFT AID: _____

OTOSCOPY: Clear bilaterally

HISTORY/IMPRESSIONS/RECOMMENDATIONS: Acoustic reflex decay was negative bilaterally at 500Hz and 1000Hz. _____

_____

_____

_____

_____

AUDIOLOGIST: _____   ASSISTANT: _____   AUDIOMETER: _____

FIGURE 1.4   Patient 1

Audiogram Interpretation Exercises

PATIENT 2

Mr. B., a 57-year-old male, was seen for an audiologic evaluation. He reported experiencing difficulty understanding speech in the presence of noise and group situations. He reported some history of noise exposure in his early 20s as a result of his career as a military sergeant. Mr. B. reported intermittent tinnitus described as high-pitched whistling in both ears. The tinnitus is bothersome only at night when it is quiet. He stated that during this time the tinnitus is not affecting his quality of life. The remainder of his audiologic, otologic, and medical history is negative. This patient reported having excellent health and does not take medication at this time. There is no family history of hearing loss. (See Figure 1.5.)

1. What is the type, degree, and audiometric configuration of the hearing loss in each ear?

2. Calculate the three-frequency pure tone average in each ear.

3. Why is the PTA not a sufficient measure of communication abilities?

4. Why was the interoctave of 750 Hz tested in each ear?

5. What do the immitance results suggest about the middle-ear status?

6. Describe the ipsilateral and contralateral acoustic reflexes in each ear.

7. What are four audiologic recommendations that you would make for this patient?

NAME: Patient 2   AGE/DATE OF BIRTH: 57 y/o

REFERRED BY: MEDICAL RECORD #:

TEST INTERVAL: DATE OF TEST:

PURE TONE AUDIOMETRY (RE: ANSI 1996)

KEY:

LEFT	STIMULUS	RIGHT
X	AIR	O
☐	AIR - MASK	△
>	BONE	<
]	BONE - MASK	[
↘	NO RESPONSE	✓
L	AIDED SOUND FIELD	R
	SOUND FIELD = S	

TEST TYPE
- STANDARD CAE
- PLAY
- COR/VRA
- BOA

TRANSDUCER
- INSERT
- CIRCUMAURAL
- SOUND FIELD

RELIABILITY
- EXCELLENT
- GOOD
- FAIR
- POOR

BOOTH
- #1
- #2 (PEDS)
- #3
- #4 COCH IMPLANT

TYMPANOMETRY (226 Hz)

EAR	LEFT	RIGHT
STATIC ADMITTANCE (mm H₂O)		
TYMP PEAK PRESSURE (DaPa)		
TYMP WIDTH (DaPa)		
EAR CANAL VOLUME cm³	.85	.87

CONTRA	.5k Hz	1k Hz	2k Hz	4k Hz	IPSI	.5k Hz	1k Hz	2k Hz	4k Hz
Right (AD) (phone ear)	90	85	90	100	AD (probe ear)	90	90	95	
Left (AS) (phone ear)	90	85	90	100	AS (probe ear)	90	90	95	

MIDDLE EAR ANALYZER _____

SPEECH AUDIOMETRY

	PTA	SRT/SAT	Speech Recognition	Speech Recognition	MCL	UCL
RIGHT (AD)	40		96 %	80 dBHL	%	65	100+
Masking						
LEFT (AS)	40		96%	80 dBHL	%	65	100+
Masking						

	MLV ☐	CD/tape ☒	W-22 ☐	WIPI ☐	PBK ☐	SPECIAL: NU #6	SPECIAL:
SOUND FIELD	55dBHL* 84 %		%				
RIGHT AIDED	%		%				
LEFT AIDED	%		%				
BINAURAL	%		%				

OTOACOUSTIC EMISSIONS (OAEs)

EMISSION TYPE USED	TEST TYPE PERFORMED
Transient	OAE Complete
Distortion Product	OAE Screening
OAE results:	
Right Ear	
Left Ear	

OAE UNIT _____

HEARING AID INFORMATION

RIGHT AID: _____

LEFT AID: _____

OTOSCOPY: Clear bilaterally

*With S/N ratio of 0dB

HISTORY/IMPRESSIONS/RECOMMENDATIONS: Acoustic reflex decay was negative at 500Hz and 1000 Hz bilaterally.

AUDIOLOGIST: _____ ASSISTANT: _____ AUDIOMETER: _____

FIGURE 1.5 Patient 2

PATIENT 3

Ms. L., a 44-year-old female, was seen for an audiologic evaluation due to complaints of decreased hearing bilaterally. She stated that the hearing loss appears to be worse in the right ear. Ms. L. stated that her maternal grandmother had a hearing loss for as long as she could remember and that she has worn bilateral hearing aids. There were no other family members with hearing loss to her knowledge. Ms. L. stated that she noticed the hearing loss after she gave birth to her second child. The audiologist noted that the whites of Ms. L.'s eyes appeared to have a bluish tint. Otoscopy revealed that the cone of light was absent in the right and left ears. She stated that she has fewer problems understanding speech in noise conditions as compared to quiet environments. The remainder of her otologic, audiologic, and medical histories was unremarkable.

1. Describe the patient's hearing sensitivity in each ear. (See Figure 1.6.)

2. At which frequencies was masking done for bone conduction? Why was masking done at these frequencies?

3. What is the significance of the decreased bone conduction at threshold 2000 Hz bilaterally?

4. What type of word recognition results were obtained for this patient at 40 dB SL re: SRT?

5. What would be the expected immittance results in each ear?

6. Would you expect otoacoustic emissions (OAEs) in each ear? Why or why not?

7. What is the possible etiology of the hearing loss?

8. What audiologic signs suggest the etiology you identified?

9. What audiologic recommendations would you make?

NAME: Patient 3　　　　　　　　　　　AGE/DATE OF BIRTH: __44 y/o__

REFERRED BY: _____　MEDICAL RECORD #: _____

TEST INTERVAL: _____　DATE OF TEST: _____

PURE TONE AUDIOMETRY (RE: ANSI 1996)

KEY:		
LEFT	**STIMULUS**	**RIGHT**
X	AIR	O
☐	AIR - MASK	Δ
>	BONE	<
]	BONE - MASK	[
↘	NO RESPONSE	↙
L	AIDED SOUND FIELD	R
	SOUND FIELD = **S**	

TEST TYPE
- STANDARD CAE
- PLAY
- COR/VRA
- BOA

TRANSDUCER
- INSERT
- CIRCUMAURAL
- SOUND FIELD

RELIABILITY
- EXCELLENT
- GOOD
- FAIR
- POOR

BOOTH
- #1
- #2 (PEDS)
- #3
- #4 COCH IMPLANT

TYMPANOMETRY (226 Hz)

EAR	LEFT	RIGHT
STATIC ADMITTANCE (mm H₂O)		
TYMP PEAK PRESSURE (DaPa)		
TYMP WIDTH (DaPa)		
EAR CANAL VOLUME cm³		

LEFT　　　RIGHT

Admittance

Pressure　　　Pressure

CONTRA	5k Hz	1k Hz	2k Hz	4k Hz	IPSI	.5k Hz	1k Hz	2k Hz	4k Hz
Right (AD) (phone ear)					AD (probe ear)				
Left (AS) (phone ear)					AS (probe ear)				

MIDDLE EAR ANALYZER _____

SPEECH AUDIOMETRY

	PTA	SRT/SAT	Speech Recognition		Speech Recognition		MCL	UCL
RIGHT (AD)		50	96 %	90 / 70	%			
Masking								
LEFT (AS)		50	92 %	90 / 70	%			
Masking								

MLV ☐	CD/tape ☒	W-22 ☐	WIPI ☐	PBK ☐	SPECIAL: NU #6	SPECIAL:
SOUND FIELD		%			%	
RIGHT AIDED		%			%	
LEFT AIDED		%			%	
BINAURAL		%			%	

OTOACOUSTIC EMISSIONS (OAEs)

EMISSION TYPE USED	TEST TYPE PERFORMED
Transient	OAE Complete
Distortion Product	OAE Screening
OAE results:	
Right Ear	
Left Ear	

OAE UNIT _____

HEARING AID INFORMATION

RIGHT AID: _____

LEFT AID: _____

OTOSCOPY: _____

HISTORY/IMPRESSIONS/RECOMMENDATIONS: _____

_____

_____

_____

_____

_____

AUDIOLOGIST: _____　ASSISTANT: _____　AUDIOMETER: _____

FIGURE 1.6　Patient 3

Audiogram Interpretation Exercises

PATIENT 4

Ms. S., 35-year-old female, was seen for an audiologic evaluation. She was referred by her endocrinologist. Ms. S. has type I diabetes, which was diagnosed in her teenage years. She has been insulin-dependent for the last 20 years. S. has reported experiencing high blood glucose levels (>300 mg/100 ml) for the last several weeks. She reported that in the last two months she has been experiencing difficulty hearing. In addition, she has high-pitched constant tinnitus that appears to be in the midline of her head. The tinnitus has been present for about two years. There is no history of hearing loss in her family. S. has some vision problems as a result of diabetes (e.g., diabetic retinopathy) in both eyes, for which she is under ophthalmologic care. She uses magnification to help with her vision loss. (See Figure 1.7.)

1. Describe diabetes's potential impact on the auditory mechanism.

2. Describe the pure tone thresholds in each ear in audiogram 1.

3. Describe the speech audiometric results in each ear.

4. Are the pure tone averages and SRT results in agreement in each ear?

5. What do the immittance results suggest about middle-ear function?

6. Describe otoacoustic emission (OAE) screening data.

Follow-Up Audiogram for Patient S

S. went into a diabetic coma one month ago. When she came out of the coma, S. stated that her hearing sensitivity seemed to be poorer in both ears, and she is experiencing dysequilibrium. A follow-up audiogram was conducted three months after S.'s initial audiological evaluation. It revealed decreased in hearing sensitivity especially for the high frequencies. In addition, S. reported that tinnitus is continuous and has gotten louder since her previous evaluation two months ago. Her blood glucose levels continue to be very high (400 mg/100 ml) despite several changes in her insulin levels. (See Figure 1.8.)

7. Describe the changes in pure tone and speech results since S.'s previous audiogram 1.

8. What follow-up testing should be done due to the patient's report of dysequilibrium?

9. What audiologic recommendations would you make for this patient?

NAME: Patient 4

REFERRED BY: _____

TEST INTERVAL: _____

sloping to mild HL @ high freqs

AGE/DATE OF BIRTH: 35 y/o

MEDICAL RECORD #: _____

DATE OF TEST: _____

PURE TONE AUDIOMETRY (RE: ANSI 1996)

TYMPANOMETRY (226 Hz)

EAR	LEFT	RIGHT
STATIC ADMITTANCE (mm H₂O)		
TYMP PEAK PRESSURE (DaPa)		
TYMP WIDTH (DaPa)		
EAR CANAL VOLUME cm³	1.1	1.0

LEFT   RIGHT

Admittance

Pressure   Pressure

CONTRA	.5k Hz	1k Hz	2k Hz	4k Hz	IPSI	.5k Hz	1k Hz	2k Hz	4k Hz
Right (AD) (phone ear)	85	80	85	90	AD (probe ear)	85	90	90	
Left (AS) (phone ear)	85	90	95	85	AS (probe ear)	85	90	90	

MIDDLE EAR ANALYZER _____

SPEECH AUDIOMETRY

	PTA	SRT/SAT	Speech Recognition	Speech Recognition	MCL	UCL
RIGHT (AD)	13	15	100%	55 dBHL / %		
Masking						
LEFT (AS)	13	15	100%	55 dBHL / %		
Masking						

MLV ☐	CD/tape ☒	W-22 ☐	WIPI ☐	PBK ☐	SPECIAL: NU #6	SPECIAL:
SOUND FIELD		%		%		
RIGHT AIDED		%		%		
LEFT AIDED		%		%		
BINAURAL		%		%		

OTOACOUSTIC EMISSIONS (OAEs)

EMISSION TYPE USED	TEST TYPE PERFORMED
Transient	OAE Complete
Distortion Product	☒ OAE Screening

OAE results:

Right Ear	Present
Left Ear	Present

OAE UNIT _____

HEARING AID INFORMATION

RIGHT AID: _____

LEFT AID: _____

OTOSCOPY: _____

HISTORY/IMPRESSIONS/RECOMMENDATIONS: Acoustic Reflex decay was negative bilaterally at 500Hz and 1000Hz. Tinnitus bilaterally

_____

_____

_____

_____

_____

AUDIOLOGIST: _____   ASSISTANT: _____   AUDIOMETER: _____

FIGURE 1.7 Patient 4

Audiogram Interpretation Exercises

NAME: Patient 4-Follow up   AGE/DATE OF BIRTH: 35 y/o

REFERRED BY: _____   MEDICAL RECORD #: _____

TEST INTERVAL: _____   DATE OF TEST: _____

PURE TONE AUDIOMETRY (RE: ANSI 1996)

KEY:

	STIMULUS	
LEFT		RIGHT
X	AIR	O
☐	AIR - MASK	△
>	BONE	<
]	BONE - MASK	[
↘	NO RESPONSE	✓
L	AIDED SOUND FIELD	R
	SOUND FIELD = S	

TEST TYPE

STANDARD CAE	
PLAY	
COR/VRA	
BOA	

TRANSDUCER

INSERT	
CIRCUMAURAL	
SOUND FIELD	

RELIABILITY

EXCELLENT	
GOOD	
FAIR	
POOR	

BOOTH

#1	
#2 (PEDS)	
#3	
#4 COCH IMPLANT	

TYMPANOMETRY (226 Hz)

EAR	LEFT	RIGHT
STATIC ADMITTANCE (mm H₂O)		
TYMP PEAK PRESSURE (DaPa)		
TYMP WIDTH (DaPa)		
EAR CANAL VOLUME cm³	.89	.93

LEFT   RIGHT

Admittance

Pressure   Pressure

CONTRA	5k Hz	1k Hz	2k Hz	4k Hz	IPSI	5k Hz	1k Hz	2k Hz	4k Hz
Right (AD) (phone ear)	85	80	85	90	AD (probe ear)	85	90	90	
Left (AS) (phone ear)	85	90	95	85	AS (probe ear)	85	90	90	

MIDDLE EAR ANALYZER _____

SPEECH AUDIOMETRY

	PTA	SRT / SAT	Speech Recognition		Speech Recognition	MCL	UCL
RIGHT (AD)	13	15	88 %	55 dBHL	%		
Masking							
LEFT (AS)	13	15	84 %	55 dBHL	%		
Masking							

MLV ☐	CD/tape ☒	W-22 ☒	WIPI ☐	PBK ☐	SPECIAL:	SPECIAL:
SOUND FIELD			%		%	
RIGHT AIDED			%		%	
LEFT AIDED			%		%	
BINAURAL			%		%	

OTOACOUSTIC EMISSIONS (OAEs)

EMISSION TYPE USED	TEST TYPE PERFORMED
Transient	OAE Complete
Distortion Product ☒	OAE Screening

OAE results:

Right Ear	Absent
Left Ear	Absent

OAE UNIT _____

HEARING AID INFORMATION

RIGHT AID: _____

LEFT AID: _____

OTOSCOPY: _____

HISTORY/IMPRESSIONS/RECOMMENDATIONS: Acoustic Reflex decay was negative bilaterally at 500Hz and 1000Hz. Tinnitus bilaterally

_____

_____

_____

_____

AUDIOLOGIST: _____   ASSISTANT: _____   AUDIOMETER: _____

FIGURE 1.8 Patient 4 Follow-Up

PATIENT 5

Ms. G., a 48-year-old female, was seen for a baseline audiogram prior to initiation of chemotherapy. She was diagnosed with breast cancer that has metastasized to the brain. At the time of this initial evaluation, Ms. G. did not report any problems with her hearing. Her history was negative for balance problems or tinnitus. Ms. G. was referred for an audiologic evaluation by her oncologist. She will be treated with cisplatin, which is known to be ototoxic. The patient's hearing sensitivity will be monitored on a weekly basis during her five weeks of chemotherapy and at one month and three months following the cessation of chemotherapy treatment. (See Figures 1.9a–1.9g.)

Audiogram 1

1. Describe the patient's hearing sensitivity in each ear.

2. Describe the patient's word recognition ability.

3. What do the immittance results in each ear suggest?

4. Describe the OAE results for each ear.

Serial Audiograms 2–4

1. Has the patient's hearing sensitivity changed since her baseline audiogram?

2. What additional tests would you conduct to see whether there are any ototoxic effects on the auditory mechanism?

Audiogram 5 (completed 4 and 5 weeks after the cessation of chemotherapy treatment)

1. Describe the patient's hearing sensitivity.

2. Describe the patient's OAEs.

3. What may be the reason for the OAE results?

4. Describe the patient's word recognition scores.

5. Are there significant differences between audiograms 6 and 7, taken at one month and three months respectively, as compared to audiograms 4 and 5?

6. What recommendations would you make for this patient?

Audiogram Interpretation Exercises

NAME: Patient 5   AGE/DATE OF BIRTH: _____

REFERRED BY: _____   MEDICAL RECORD #: _____

TEST INTERVAL: Week 1 _____   DATE OF TEST: _____

PURE TONE AUDIOMETRY (RE: ANSI 1996)

KEY:		
LEFT	STIMULUS	RIGHT
X	AIR	O
▢	AIR - MASK	Δ
>	BONE	<
]	BONE - MASK	[
↘	NO RESPONSE	✓
L	AIDED SOUND FIELD	R
	SOUND FIELD = S	

TEST TYPE
- STANDARD CAE
- PLAY
- COR/VRA
- BOA

TRANSDUCER
- INSERT
- CIRCUMAURAL
- SOUND FIELD

RELIABILITY
- EXCELLENT
- GOOD
- FAIR
- POOR

BOOTH
- #1
- #2 (PEDS)
- #3
- #4 COCH IMPLANT

TYMPANOMETRY (226 Hz)

EAR	LEFT	RIGHT
STATIC ADMITTANCE (mm H$_2$O)		
TYMP PEAK PRESSURE (DaPa)		
TYMP WIDTH (DaPa)		
EAR CANAL VOLUME cm^3	.74	.68

LEFT   Admittance   RIGHT

Pressure   Pressure

	CONTRA	.5k Hz	1k Hz	2k Hz	4k Hz	IPSI	.5k Hz	1k Hz	2k Hz	4k Hz
Right (AD) (phone ear)		90	90	95	85	AD (probe ear)	95	95	95	
Left (AS) (phone ear)		95	90	85	90	AS (probe ear)	90	90	90	

MIDDLE EAR ANALYZER _____

SPEECH AUDIOMETRY

	PTA	SRT/SAT	Speech Recognition		Speech Recognition	MCL	UCL
RIGHT (AD)		0	100 %	40 dBHL	%		
Masking							
LEFT (AS)		0	100 %	40 dBHL	%		
Masking							

MLV ☐	CD/tape ☒	W-22 ☐	WIPI ☐	PBK ☐	SPECIAL: NU #6	SPECIAL:
SOUND FIELD		%			%	
RIGHT AIDED		%			%	
LEFT AIDED		%			%	
BINAURAL		%			%	

OTOACOUSTIC EMISSIONS (OAEs)

EMISSION TYPE USED	TEST TYPE PERFORMED
☒ Transient	OAE Complete
Distortion Product	☒ OAE Screening

OAE results:

Right Ear   Present

Left Ear   Present

OAE UNIT _____

HEARING AID INFORMATION

RIGHT AID: _____

LEFT AID: _____

OTOSCOPY: _____

HISTORY/IMPRESSIONS/RECOMMENDATIONS: Acoustic Reflex Decay was negative bilaterally at 500Hz and 1000Hz _____

_____

_____

_____

_____

_____

AUDIOLOGIST: _____   ASSISTANT: _____   AUDIOMETER: _____

FIGURE 1.9A   Patient 5, Audiogram 1

NAME: Client 5

AGE/DATE OF BIRTH: _____

REFERRED BY: _____

MEDICAL RECORD #: _____

TEST INTERVAL: Baseline

DATE OF TEST: _____

PURE TONE AUDIOMETRY (RE: ANSI 1996)

KEY:		
LEFT	STIMULUS	RIGHT
X	AIR	O
□	AIR - MASK	△
>	BONE	<
]	BONE - MASK	[
↘	NO RESPONSE	↙
L	AIDED SOUND FIELD	R
	SOUND FIELD = S	

TEST TYPE
STANDARD CAE
PLAY
COR/VRA
BOA

TRANSDUCER
INSERT
CIRCUMAURAL
SOUND FIELD

RELIABILITY
EXCELLENT
GOOD
FAIR
POOR

BOOTH
#1
#2 (PEDS)
#3
#4 COCH IMPLANT

TYMPANOMETRY (226 Hz)

EAR	LEFT	RIGHT
STATIC ADMITTANCE (mm H₂O)		
TYMP PEAK PRESSURE (DaPa)		
TYMP WIDTH (DaPa)		
EAR CANAL VOLUME cm³	.74	.68

LEFT   RIGHT
Admittance
Pressure   Pressure

CONTRA	5k Hz	1k Hz	2k Hz	4k Hz	IPSI	5k Hz	1k Hz	2k Hz	4k Hz
Right (AD) (phone ear)	90	90	95	85	AD (probe ear)	95	95	95	
Left (AS) (phone ear)	95	90	85	90	AS (probe ear)	90	90	90	

MIDDLE EAR ANALYZER _____

SPEECH AUDIOMETRY

	PTA	SRT/ SAT	Speech Recognition		Speech Recognition		MCL	UCL
RIGHT (AD) Masking		0	100 %	40 dBHL	%			
LEFT (AS) Masking		0	100 %	40 dBHL	%			

MLV □	CD/tape ☒	W-22 □	WIPI □	PBK □	SPECIAL: NU #6	SPECIAL:
SOUND FIELD		%			%	
RIGHT AIDED		%			%	
LEFT AIDED		%			%	
BINAURAL		%			%	

OTOACOUSTIC EMISSIONS (OAEs)

EMISSION TYPE USED	TEST TYPE PERFORMED
☒ Transient	OAE Complete
Distortion Product	☒ OAE Screening

OAE results:

Right Ear Present

Left Ear Present

OAE UNIT _____

HEARING AID INFORMATION

RIGHT AID: _____

LEFT AID: _____

OTOSCOPY: _____

HISTORY/IMPRESSIONS/RECOMMENDATIONS: Acoustic Reflex Decay was negative bilaterally at 500Hz and 1000Hz _____

_____

_____

_____

_____

AUDIOLOGIST: _____ ASSISTANT: _____ AUDIOMETER: _____

FIGURE 1.9B Patient 5, Audiogram 2

NAME: Patient 5 AGE/DATE OF BIRTH: _____

REFERRED BY: _____ MEDICAL RECORD #: _____

TEST INTERVAL: Week 2 DATE OF TEST: _____

PURE TONE AUDIOMETRY (RE: ANSI 1996)

KEY:		
LEFT	STIMULUS	RIGHT
X	AIR	O
□	AIR - MASK	Δ
>	BONE	<
]	BONE - MASK	[
↘	NO RESPONSE	↙
	AIDED	√
L	SOUND FIELD	R
	SOUND FIELD = S	

TEST TYPE
- STANDARD CAE
- PLAY
- COR/VRA
- BOA

TRANSDUCER
- INSERT
- CIRCUMAURAL
- SOUND FIELD

RELIABILITY
- EXCELLENT
- GOOD
- FAIR
- POOR

BOOTH
- #1
- #2 (PEDS)
- #3
- #4 COCH IMPLANT

TYMPANOMETRY (226 Hz)

EAR	LEFT	RIGHT
STATIC ADMITTANCE (mm H₂O)		
TYMP PEAK PRESSURE (DaPa)		
TYMP WIDTH (DaPa)		
EAR CANAL VOLUME cm³	.74	.68

LEFT   Pressure

RIGHT   Pressure

Admittance

CONTRA	.5k Hz	1k Hz	2k Hz	4k Hz	IPSI	.5k Hz	1k Hz	2k Hz	4k Hz
Right (AD) (phone ear)	90	90	95	85	AD (probe ear)	95	95	95	
Left (AS) (phone ear)	95	90	85	90	AS (probe ear)	90	90	90	

MIDDLE EAR ANALYZER _____

SPEECH AUDIOMETRY

	PTA	SRT/SAT	Speech Recognition		Speech Recognition	MCL	UCL
RIGHT (AD)		0	100 %	40 dBHL	%		
Masking							
LEFT (AS)		0	100 %	40 dBHL	%		
Masking							

MLV ☐	CD/tape ☒	W-22 ☐	WIPI ☐	PBK ☐	SPECIAL: NU #6	SPECIAL:
SOUND FIELD		%			%	
RIGHT AIDED		%			%	
LEFT AIDED		%			%	
BINAURAL		%			%	

OTOACOUSTIC EMISSIONS (OAEs)

EMISSION TYPE USED		TEST TYPE PERFORMED
☒	Transient	OAE Complete
	Distortion Product	☒ OAE Screening

OAE results:

Right Ear Present

Left Ear Present

OAE UNIT _____

HEARING AID INFORMATION

RIGHT AID: _____

LEFT AID: _____

OTOSCOPY: _____

HISTORY/IMPRESSIONS/RECOMMENDATIONS: Acoustic Reflex Decay was negative bilaterally at 500Hz and 1000Hz

_____

_____

_____

_____

_____

AUDIOLOGIST: _____ ASSISTANT: _____ AUDIOMETER: _____

FIGURE 1.9C Patient 5, Audiogram 3

NAME: Patient 5

AGE/DATE OF BIRTH: _____

REFERRED BY: _____

MEDICAL RECORD #: _____

TEST INTERVAL: Week 3

DATE OF TEST: _____

PURE TONE AUDIOMETRY (RE: ANSI 1996)

KEY:		
LEFT	STIMULUS	RIGHT
X	AIR	O
☐	AIR - MASK	△
>	BONE	<
]	BONE - MASK	[
↘	NO RESPONSE	✓
L	AIDED SOUND FIELD	R
	SOUND FIELD = S	

TEST TYPE
- STANDARD CAE
- PLAY
- COR/VRA
- BOA

TRANSDUCER
- INSERT
- CIRCUMAURAL
- SOUND FIELD

RELIABILITY
- EXCELLENT
- GOOD
- FAIR
- POOR

BOOTH
- #1
- #2 (PEDS)
- #3
- #4 COCH IMPLANT

TYMPANOMETRY (226 Hz)

EAR	LEFT	RIGHT
STATIC ADMITTANCE (mm H₂O)		
TYMP PEAK PRESSURE (DaPa)		
TYMP WIDTH (DaPa)		
EAR CANAL VOLUME cm³	.74	.68

LEFT   Admittance   RIGHT

Pressure   Pressure

CONTRA	5k Hz	1k Hz	2k Hz	4k Hz	IPSI	5k Hz	1k Hz	2k Hz	4k Hz
Right (AD) (phone ear)	90	90	95	85	AD (probe ear)	95	95	95	
Left (AS) (phone ear)	95	90	85	90	AS (probe ear)	90	90	90	

MIDDLE EAR ANALYZER _____

SPEECH AUDIOMETRY

	PTA	SRT/ SAT	Speech Recognition		Speech Recognition	MCL	UCL
RIGHT (AD)		0	100 %	40 dBHL	%		
Masking							
LEFT (AS)		0	100 %	40 dBHL	%		
Masking							

MLV ☐	CD/tape ☒	W-22 ☐	WIPI ☐	PBK ☐	SPECIAL: NU #6	SPECIAL:
SOUND FIELD		%		%		
RIGHT AIDED		%		%		
LEFT AIDED		%		%		
BINAURAL		%		%		

OTOACOUSTIC EMISSIONS (OAEs)

EMISSION TYPE USED		TEST TYPE PERFORMED
☒	Transient	OAE Complete
	Distortion Product	☒ OAE Screening

OAE results:

Right Ear   Present

Left Ear   Present

OAE UNIT _____

HEARING AID INFORMATION

RIGHT AID: _____

LEFT AID: _____

OTOSCOPY: _____

HISTORY/IMPRESSIONS/RECOMMENDATIONS: Acoustic Reflex Decay was negative bilaterally at 500Hz and 1000Hz

_____

_____

_____

_____

_____

AUDIOLOGIST: _____ ASSISTANT: _____ AUDIOMETER: _____

FIGURE 1.9D   Patient 5, Audiogram 4

Audiogram Interpretation Exercises

NAME: Patient 5　　　　　　　　　　　　AGE/DATE OF BIRTH: _____

REFERRED BY: _____　　　　　　　MEDICAL RECORD #: _____

TEST INTERVAL: Week 4-5　　　　　　　DATE OF TEST: _____

PURE TONE AUDIOMETRY (RE: ANSI 1996)

KEY:

	LEFT	STIMULUS	RIGHT	
X		AIR		O
☐		AIR - MASK		Δ
>		BONE		<
]		BONE - MASK		[
↘		NO RESPONSE		✓
L		AIDED SOUND FIELD		R
		SOUND FIELD = S		

TEST TYPE
STANDARD CAE	
PLAY	
COR/VRA	
BOA	

TRANSDUCER
INSERT	
CIRCUMAURAL	
SOUND FIELD	

RELIABILITY
EXCELLENT	
GOOD	
FAIR	
POOR	

BOOTH
#1	
#2 (PEDS)	
#3	
#4 COCH IMPLANT	

TYMPANOMETRY (226 Hz)

EAR	LEFT	RIGHT
STATIC ADMITTANCE (mm H2O)		
TYMP PEAK PRESSURE (DaPa)		
TYMP WIDTH (DaPa)		
EAR CANAL VOLUME cm³		

LEFT　　　　　　　RIGHT

Pressure　　　　　Pressure

CONTRA	.5k Hz	1k Hz	2k Hz	4k Hz	IPSI	.5k Hz	1k Hz	2k Hz	4k Hz
Right (AD) (phone ear)	90	90	95	85	AD (probe ear)	95	95	95	
Left (AS) (phone ear)	95	90	85	90	AS (probe ear)	90	90	90	

MIDDLE EAR ANALYZER _____

SPEECH AUDIOMETRY

	PTA	SRT/SAT	Speech Recognition		Speech Recognition	MCL	UCL
RIGHT (AD)		0	96 %	40 dBHL	%		
Masking							
LEFT (AS)		0	92 %	40 dBHL	%		
Masking							

MLV ☐	CD/tape ☒	W-22 ☐	WIPI ☐	PBK ☐	SPECIAL: NU #6	SPECIAL:
SOUND FIELD		%		%		
RIGHT AIDED		%		%		
LEFT AIDED		%		%		
BINAURAL		%		%		

OTOACOUSTIC EMISSIONS (OAEs)

EMISSION TYPE USED		TEST TYPE PERFORMED
☒	Transient	OAE Complete
	Distortion Product	☒ OAE Screening
	OAE results:	
Right Ear	Absent	
Left Ear	Absent	

OAE UNIT _____

HEARING AID INFORMATION

RIGHT AID: _____

LEFT AID: _____

OTOSCOPY: _____

HISTORY/IMPRESSIONS/RECOMMENDATIONS: Acoustic Reflex Decay was negative bilaterally at 500Hz and 1000Hz _____

_____

_____

_____

_____

AUDIOLOGIST: _____　　　ASSISTANT: _____　　　AUDIOMETER: _____

FIGURE 1.9E Patient 5, Audiogram 5

NAME: Patient 5

AGE/DATE OF BIRTH: _____

REFERRED BY: _____

MEDICAL RECORD #: _____

TEST INTERVAL: 1 month post treatment

DATE OF TEST: _____

PURE TONE AUDIOMETRY (RE: ANSI 1996)

KEY:

	STIMULUS	
LEFT		RIGHT
X	AIR	O
☐	AIR - MASK	Δ
>	BONE	<
]	BONE - MASK	[
↘	NO RESPONSE	✓
L	AIDED SOUND FIELD	R
	SOUND FIELD = S	

TEST TYPE
STANDARD CAE	
PLAY	
COR/VRA	
BOA	

TRANSDUCER
INSERT	
CIRCUMAURAL	
SOUND FIELD	

RELIABILITY
EXCELLENT	
GOOD	
FAIR	
POOR	

BOOTH
#1	
#2 (PEDS)	
#3	
#4 COCH IMPLANT	

TYMPANOMETRY (226 Hz)

EAR	LEFT	RIGHT
STATIC ADMITTANCE (mm H₂O)		
TYMP PEAK PRESSURE (DaPa)		
TYMP WIDTH (DaPa)		
EAR CANAL VOLUME cm³		

LEFT   Admittance   RIGHT

Pressure   Pressure

CONTRA	.5k Hz	1k Hz	2k Hz	4k Hz	IPSI	.5k Hz	1k Hz	2k Hz	4k Hz
Right (AD) (phone ear)	90	90	95	85	AD (probe ear)	95	95	95	
Left (AS) (phone ear)	95	90	85	90	AS (probe ear)	90	90	90	

MIDDLE EAR ANALYZER _____

SPEECH AUDIOMETRY

	PTA	SRT/SAT	Speech Recognition		Speech Recognition		MCL	UCL
RIGHT (AD)		0	96 %	40 dBHL	%			
Masking								
LEFT (AS)		0	92 %	40 dBHL	%			
Masking								

	MLV ☐	CD/tape ☒	W-22 ☐	WIPI ☐	PBK ☐	SPECIAL: NU #6	SPECIAL:
SOUND FIELD			%			%	
RIGHT AIDED			%			%	
LEFT AIDED			%			%	
BINAURAL			%			%	

OTOACOUSTIC EMISSIONS (OAEs)

EMISSION TYPE USED	TEST TYPE PERFORMED
☒ Transient	OAE Complete
Distortion Product	☒ OAE Screening

OAE results:

Right Ear   Absent

Left Ear   Absent

OAE UNIT _____

HEARING AID INFORMATION

RIGHT AID: _____

LEFT AID: _____

OTOSCOPY: _____

HISTORY/IMPRESSIONS/RECOMMENDATIONS: Acoustic Reflex Decay was negative bilaterally at 500Hz and 1000Hz _____

_____

_____

_____

_____

_____

AUDIOLOGIST: _____ ASSISTANT: _____ AUDIOMETER: _____

FIGURE 1.9F Patient 5, Audiogram 6

NAME: Patient 5

AGE/DATE OF BIRTH: _____

REFERRED BY: _____

MEDICAL RECORD #: _____

TEST INTERVAL: 3 months post treatment

DATE OF TEST: _____

PURE TONE AUDIOMETRY (RE: ANSI 1996)

KEY:

LEFT	STIMULUS	RIGHT
X	AIR	O
☐	AIR - MASK	Δ
>	BONE	<
]	BONE - MASK	[
↘	NO RESPONSE	↙
L	AIDED SOUND FIELD	R
	SOUND FIELD = S	

TEST TYPE
- STANDARD CAE
- PLAY
- COR/VRA
- BOA

TRANSDUCER
- INSERT
- CIRCUMAURAL
- SOUND FIELD

RELIABILITY
- EXCELLENT
- GOOD
- FAIR
- POOR

BOOTH
- #1
- #2 (PEDS)
- #3
- #4 COCH IMPLANT

TYMPANOMETRY (226 Hz)

EAR	LEFT	RIGHT
STATIC ADMITTANCE (mm H₂O)		
TYMP PEAK PRESSURE (DaPa)		
TYMP WIDTH (DaPa)		
EAR CANAL VOLUME cm³		

CONTRA	5k Hz	1k Hz	2k Hz	4k Hz	IPSI	5k Hz	1k Hz	2k Hz	4k Hz
Right (AD) (phone ear)	90	90	95	85	AD (probe ear)	95	95	95	
Left (AS) (phone ear)	95	90	85	90	AS (probe ear)	90	90	90	

MIDDLE EAR ANALYZER _____

SPEECH AUDIOMETRY

	PTA	SRT/SAT	Speech Recognition		Speech Recognition	MCL	UCL
RIGHT (AD)		0	96 %	40 dBHL	%		
Masking							
LEFT (AS)		0	92 %	40 dBHL	%		
Masking							

MLV ☐	CD/tape ☒	W-22 ☐	WIPI ☐	PBK ☐	SPECIAL: NU #6	SPECIAL:
SOUND FIELD			%		%	
RIGHT AIDED			%		%	
LEFT AIDED			%		%	
BINAURAL			%		%	

OTOACOUSTIC EMISSIONS (OAEs)

EMISSION TYPE USED		TEST TYPE PERFORMED
☒ Transient		OAE Complete
Distortion Product		☒ OAE Screening

OAE results:

Right Ear   Absent

Left Ear   Absent

OAE UNIT _____

HEARING AID INFORMATION

RIGHT AID: _____

LEFT AID: _____

OTOSCOPY: _____

HISTORY/IMPRESSIONS/RECOMMENDATIONS: Acoustic Reflex Decay was negative bilaterally at 500Hz and 1000Hz

_____

_____

_____

_____

AUDIOLOGIST: _____   ASSISTANT: _____   AUDIOMETER: _____

FIGURE 1.9G   Patient 5, Audiogram 7

PATIENT 6

Mr. C., a 23-year-old male, was seen for an audiologic evaluation following an automobile accident several weeks ago. Since the time of the
automobile accident, Mr. C. has complained of a hearing loss in the left
ear with continuous roaring tinnitus in that ear. He noted that during
the accident he was jarred around a great deal and stated that he hit the
left side of his ear and head. He also reports intermittent dizziness, especially when lying down and turning his head to the left. At the time of
the accident the patient refused medical treatment. This evaluation was
requested by his car insurance company. Prior to the accident the
patient reported no problems hearing. (See Figure 1.10.)

1. Describe the patient's hearing sensitivity in each ear.

2. Describe some of the audiometric inconsistencies.

3. What is the possible reason for the inconsistent audiometric responses
   for the left ear?

4. What are the Speech Stenger results?

5. What do you think the patient's thresholds would be in the speech
   frequencies?

6. How would you resolve the audiologic inconsistencies during the test
   situation?

7. Why do you think this person may have exhibited an exaggerated
   hearing loss?

Audiogram Interpretation Exercises

NAME: Patient 6

AGE/DATE OF BIRTH: 23 y/o

REFERRED BY: _____

MEDICAL RECORD #: _____

TEST INTERVAL: _____

DATE OF TEST: _____

PURE TONE AUDIOMETRY (RE: ANSI 1996)

KEY:

	LEFT	STIMULUS	RIGHT
X		AIR	O
□		AIR - MASK	△
>		BONE	<
]		BONE - MASK	[
↘		NO RESPONSE	✓
L		AIDED SOUND FIELD	R
		SOUND FIELD = S	

TEST TYPE
- STANDARD/CAE
- PLAY
- COR/VRA
- BOA

TRANSDUCER
- INSERT
- CIRCUMAURAL
- SOUND FIELD

RELIABILITY
- EXCELLENT
- GOOD
- FAIR
- POOR

BOOTH
- #1
- #2 (PEDS)
- #3
- #4 COCH IMPLANT

TYMPANOMETRY (226 Hz)

EAR	LEFT	RIGHT
STATIC ADMITTANCE (mm H₂O)		
TYMP PEAK PRESSURE (DaPa)		
TYMP WIDTH (DaPa)		
EAR CANAL VOLUME cm³	.98	1.0

LEFT   Pressure

RIGHT   Pressure

Admittance

CONTRA	.5k Hz	1k Hz	2k Hz	4k Hz	IPSI	.5k Hz	1k Hz	2k Hz	4k Hz
Right (AD) (phone ear)	90	95	95	90	AD (probe ear)	85	90	95	
Left (AS) (phone ear)	95	100	95	90	AS (probe ear)	85	90	95	

MIDDLE EAR ANALYZER _____

SPEECH AUDIOMETRY

	PTA	SRT SAT	Speech Recognition		Speech Recognition	MCL	UCL
RIGHT (AD)	13	0	100 %	40 dBHL	%		
Masking							
LEFT (AS)	80	20	96 %	60 dBHL	%		
Masking							

MLV □	CD/tape ☒	W-22 □	WIPI □	PBK □	SPECIAL: NU #6	SPECIAL:
SOUND FIELD		%		%		
RIGHT AIDED		%		%		
LEFT AIDED		%		%		
BINAURAL		%		%		

OTOACOUSTIC EMISSIONS (OAEs)

EMISSION TYPE USED	TEST TYPE PERFORMED
☒ Transient	OAE Complete
Distortion Product	☒ OAE Screening
OAE results:	

Right Ear   Present

Left Ear   Present

OAE UNIT _____

HEARING AID INFORMATION

RIGHT AID: _____

LEFT AID: _____

OTOSCOPY: _____

HISTORY/IMPRESSIONS/RECOMMENDATIONS: Acoustic reflex decay was negative bilaterally at 500Hz and 1000 Hz.

Speech stenger was positive.

_____

_____

_____

_____

AUDIOLOGIST: _____ ASSISTANT: _____ AUDIOMETER: _____

FIGURE 1.10 Patient 6

PATIENT 7

Dr. A. is a 58-year-old male physician. About one week ago, he began experiencing vertigo, sudden hearing loss, aural fullness, and roaring tinnitus in both ears. He has been incapacitated since that time due to vertigo, which has resulted in an inability to drive and function in his complex job. Dr. A. is very depressed due to his hearing loss and tinnitus. His wife, who accompanied him to the evaluation, stated that Dr. A. has not left the house since the onset of the auditory problems. He is fearful of falling due to the vertigo. Dr. A.'s primary care physician gave him Antivert to help suppress the vertigo. Dr. A. has not slept due to the annoyance of the tinnitus and vertigo. (See Figure 1.11.)

1. What is the type, degree, and audiometric configuration of hearing loss?

2. What is the pure tone average in each ear?

3. Describe the speech recognition scores in each ear.

4. What are the results for OAEs in each ear? Is this consistent with the audiogram?

5. What is the possible etiology of hearing loss in both ears?

6. What additional tests should be recommended?

7. What are some audiologic rehabilitation recommendations for this patient?

PURE TONE AUDIOMETRY (RE: ANSI 1996)

KEY:

	LEFT	Stimulus	RIGHT
	X	AIR	O
	☐	AIR - MASK	Δ
	>	BONE	<
	]	BONE - MASK	[
	↘	NO RESPONSE	✓
	L	AIDED SOUND FIELD	R
		SOUND FIELD = S	

TEST TYPE
STANDARD CAE	
PLAY	
COR/VRA	
BOA	

TRANSDUCER
INSERT	
CIRCUMAURAL	
SOUND FIELD	

RELIABILITY
EXCELLENT	
GOOD	
FAIR	
POOR	

BOOTH
#1	
#2 (PEDS)	
#3	
#4 COCH IMPLANT	

TYMPANOMETRY (226 Hz)

EAR	LEFT	RIGHT
STATIC ADMITTANCE (mm H_2O)		
TYMP PEAK PRESSURE (DaPa)		
TYMP WIDTH (DaPa)		
EAR CANAL VOLUME cm^3		

LEFT — Pressure   RIGHT — Pressure   Admittance

CONTRA	5k Hz	1k Hz	2k Hz	4k Hz	IPSI	.5k Hz	1k Hz	2k Hz	4k Hz
Right (AD) (phone ear)	95	100	100	105	AD (probe ear)	95	95	100	
Left (AS) (phone ear)	95	95	95	90	AS (probe ear)	90	90	90	

MIDDLE EAR ANALYZER _____

SPEECH AUDIOMETRY

	PTA	SRT/SAT	Speech Recognition		Speech Recognition		MCL	UCL
RIGHT (AD)		45	72 %	75	%		65	90
Masking								
LEFT (AS)		45	76 %	75	%		65	90
Masking								

	MLV ☒	CD/tape ☐	W-22 ☐	WIPI ☐	PBK ☐	SPECIAL:	SPECIAL:
SOUND FIELD			%		%		
RIGHT AIDED			%		%		
LEFT AIDED			%		%		
BINAURAL			%		%		

OTOACOUSTIC EMISSIONS (OAEs)

EMISSION TYPE USED		TEST TYPE PERFORMED	
Transient		☒	OAE Complete
☒	Distortion Product		OAE Screening
OAE results:			
Right Ear	Absent		
Left Ear	Absent		

OAE UNIT _____

HEARING AID INFORMATION

RIGHT AID: _____

LEFT AID: _____

OTOSCOPY: _____

HISTORY/IMPRESSIONS/RECOMMENDATIONS: Moderately severe (250-500Hz) rising to moderate 1000Hz-4000Hz with a gradually sloping loss 6000Hz-8000Hz sensorineural hearing loss bilaterally. _____

_____

_____

_____

AUDIOLOGIST: _____   ASSISTANT: _____   AUDIOMETER: _____

FIGURE 1.11 Patient 7

PATIENT 8

Mr. H., a 48-year-old male, was seen for an initial audiologic evaluation on referral by an ENT. His main complaint was that he has a hearing loss in his left ear. He also reported high-pitched tinnitus in his left ear. He reported no hearing difficulties in his right ear. He reported that he is very healthy. Mr. H.'s medical history was unremarkable. (See Figure 1.12.)

1. What concerns do you have about the audiologic test results?

2. What is the possible etiology of the unilateral sensorineural hearing loss?

3. What other tests and recommendations would you make?

4. What tests might the ENT physician recommend?

5. What are the possible options for the patient if a VIII nerve tumor is present?

NAME: Patient 8   **AGE/DATE OF BIRTH:** 48 y/o

REFERRED BY: _____   **MEDICAL RECORD #:** _____

TEST INTERVAL: _____   **DATE OF TEST:** _____

PURE TONE AUDIOMETRY (RE: ANSI 1996)

KEY:

LEFT	Stimulus	RIGHT
X	AIR	O
☐	AIR - MASK	Δ
>	BONE	<
]	BONE - MASK	[
↘	NO RESPONSE	✓
L	AIDED SOUND FIELD	R
	SOUND FIELD = S	

TEST TYPE

STANDARD CAE	
PLAY	
COR/VRA	
BOA	

TRANSDUCER

INSERT	
CIRCUMAURAL	
SOUND FIELD	

RELIABILITY

EXCELLENT	
GOOD	
FAIR	
POOR	

BOOTH

#1	
#2 (PEDS)	
#3	
#4 COCH IMPLANT	

TYMPANOMETRY (226 Hz)

EAR	LEFT	RIGHT
STATIC ADMITTANCE (mm H₂O)		
TYMP PEAK PRESSURE (DaPa)		
TYMP WIDTH (DaPa)		
EAR CANAL VOLUME cm³	1.0	1.2

LEFT   RIGHT

Pressure   Pressure

CONTRA	5k Hz	1k Hz	2k Hz	4k Hz	IPSI	5k Hz	1k Hz	2k Hz	4k Hz
Right (AD) (phone ear)	80	80	85	90	AD (probe ear)	80	80	80	
Left (AS) (phone ear)	NR	NR	NR	NR	AS (probe ear)	NR	NR	NR	

MIDDLE EAR ANALYZER _____

SPEECH AUDIOMETRY

	PTA	SRT/SAT	Speech Recognition	Speech Recognition	MCL	UCL
RIGHT (AD)	10	100 %	50	%		
Masking						
LEFT (AS)	40	56 %	80 / 60	40 %	90 / 70	
Masking						

MLV ☐	CD/tape ☐	W-22 ☐	WIPI ☐	PBK ☐	SPECIAL:	SPECIAL:
SOUND FIELD			%		%	
RIGHT AIDED			%		%	
LEFT AIDED			%		%	
BINAURAL			%		%	

OTOACOUSTIC EMISSIONS (OAEs)

EMISSION TYPE USED	TEST TYPE PERFORMED
Transient	OAE Complete
Distortion Product	OAE Screening

OAE results:

Right Ear	Present
Left Ear	Absent

OAE UNIT _____

HEARING AID INFORMATION

RIGHT AID: _____

LEFT AID: _____

OTOSCOPY: _____

HISTORY/IMPRESSIONS/RECOMMENDATIONS: Acoustic reflex decay was negative 500Hz at 500Hz and 1000Hz in the right ear.

_____

_____

_____

_____

_____

AUDIOLOGIST: _____   **ASSISTANT:** _____   **AUDIOMETER:** _____

FIGURE 1.12 Patient 8

Ms. D., a 30-year-old female, was referred for an audiologic evaluation by her neurologist, whom she has been seeing her for one month. D. has been experiencing tingling sensations in her extremities for about six months. She also experiences intermittent double vision, and her color vision seems dimmed. In the last month, D. has been experiencing low-pitched intermittent tinnitus and dizziness. Prior to the onset of these symptoms, D. was in excellent health. There is no family history of hearing loss, but there is a history of multiple sclerosis on the maternal side of the family. Both of her brothers have multiple sclerosis. (See Figure 1.13.)

1. What concerns you about the information attained in the case history?

2. Describe the hearing sensitivity in each ear.

3. Why do you think the acoustic reflexes are not measurable in the right ear for contralateral and ipsilateral stimulation?

4. Describe the ABR results.

5. What is the possible etiology of the hearing loss?

NAME: Patient 9

AGE/DATE OF BIRTH: _____

REFERRED BY: _____

MEDICAL RECORD #: _____

TEST INTERVAL: _____

DATE OF TEST: _____

PURE TONE AUDIOMETRY (RE: ANSI 1996)

KEY:

LEFT	Stimulus	RIGHT
X	AIR	O
☐	AIR - MASK	∆
>	BONE	<
]	BONE - MASK	[
↘	NO RESPONSE	✓
L	AIDED SOUND FIELD	R
	SOUND FIELD = S	

TEST TYPE

STANDARD CAE
PLAY
COR/VRA
BOA

TRANSDUCER

INSERT
CIRCUMAURAL
SOUND FIELD

RELIABILITY

EXCELLENT
GOOD
FAIR
POOR

BOOTH

#1
#2 (PEDS)
#3
#4 COCH IMPLANT

TYMPANOMETRY (226 Hz)

EAR	LEFT	RIGHT
STATIC ADMITTANCE (mm H$_2$O)		
TYMP PEAK PRESSURE (DaPa)		
TYMP WIDTH (DaPa)		
EAR CANAL VOLUME cm^3	.54	.72

LEFT   Pressure

RIGHT   Pressure

CONTRA	.5k Hz	1k Hz	2k Hz	4k Hz	IPSI	.5k Hz	1k Hz	2k Hz	4k Hz
Right (AD) (phone ear)	NR	NR	NR	NR	AD (probe ear)	NR	NR	NR	
Left (AS) (phone ear)	NR	NR	NR	NR	AS (probe ear)	90	85	80	

MIDDLE EAR ANALYZER _____

SPEECH AUDIOMETRY

	PTA	SRT/SAT	Speech Recognition	Speech Recognition	MCL	UCL
RIGHT (AD)	66	65	72 %	%		
Masking						
LEFT (AS)	10	5	100%	%		
Masking						

MLV ☒	CD/tape ☐	W-22 ☐	WIPI ☐	PBK ☐	SPECIAL:	SPECIAL:
SOUND FIELD			%		%	
RIGHT AIDED			%		%	
LEFT AIDED			%		%	
BINAURAL			%		%	

OTOACOUSTIC EMISSIONS (OAEs)

EMISSION TYPE USED	TEST TYPE PERFORMED
Transient	OAE Complete
Distortion Product	OAE Screening
OAE results:	
Right Ear Absent	
Left Ear Present	

OAE UNIT _____

HEARING AID INFORMATION

RIGHT AID: _____

LEFT AID: _____

OTOSCOPY: _____

HISTORY/IMPRESSIONS/RECOMMENDATIONS: ABR was normal in the left ear waves I-V ertr not present in the right ear. _____

_____

_____

_____

_____

AUDIOLOGIST: _____   ASSISTANT: _____   AUDIOMETER: _____

FIGURE 1.13   Patient 9

K., a 38-year old female, was referred by her ophthalmologist for an audiologic evaluation. K. was diagnosed recently with retinitis pigmentosa. K. began having visual problems approximately two years ago. K. has noticed that she is experiencing a decrease in her central visual fields. Over the past year, K. has noticed a decrease in her hearing sensitivity. There is no family history of hearing loss. K. is a social worker who specializes in working with individuals with hearing loss and their families. The remainder of K.'s medical history is unremarkable. (See Figure 1.14.)

1. Describe the hearing loss.

2. Describe the patient's word recognition ability in each ear.

3. What might be the etiology of the hearing loss and why?

4. What recommendations would you make for this patient?

NAME: Patient 10   AGE/DATE OF BIRTH: 38 y/o

REFERRED BY: _____   MEDICAL RECORD #: _____

TEST INTERVAL: _____   DATE OF TEST: _____

PURE TONE AUDIOMETRY (RE: ANSI 1996)

KEY:

LEFT	STIMULUS	RIGHT
X	AIR	O
☐	AIR - MASK	Δ
>	BONE	<
]	BONE - MASK	[
↓	NO RESPONSE	✓
L	AIDED SOUND FIELD	R
	SOUND FIELD = S	

TEST TYPE
STANDARD CAE
PLAY
COR/VRA
BOA

TRANSDUCER
INSERT
CIRCUMAURAL
SOUND FIELD

RELIABILITY
EXCELLENT
GOOD
FAIR
POOR

BOOTH
#1
#2 (PEDS)
#3
#4 COCH IMPLANT

TYMPANOMETRY (226 Hz)

EAR	LEFT	RIGHT
STATIC ADMITTANCE (mm H₂O)		
TYMP PEAK PRESSURE (DaPa)		
TYMP WIDTH (DaPa)		
EAR CANAL VOLUME cm³		

LEFT   RIGHT

Pressure   Pressure

CONTRA	.5k Hz	1k Hz	2k Hz	4k Hz	IPSI	.5k Hz	1k Hz	2k Hz	4k Hz
Right (AD) (phone ear)	85	80	85	80	AD (probe ear)	90	95	90	
Left (AS) (phone ear)	80	80	80	NR	AS (probe ear)	85	80	80	

MIDDLE EAR ANALYZER _____

SPEECH AUDIOMETRY

	PTA	SRT/SAT	Speech Recognition	Speech Recognition	MCL	UCL
RIGHT (AD)	40	96 %	80	%		
Masking			40			
LEFT (AS)	40	96 %	80	%		
Masking			40			

MLV ☐	CD/tape ☐	W-22 ☐	WIPI ☐	PBK ☐	SPECIAL:		SPECIAL:
SOUND FIELD			%		%		
RIGHT AIDED			%		%		
LEFT AIDED			%		%		
BINAURAL			%		%		

OTOACOUSTIC EMISSIONS (OAEs)

EMISSION TYPE USED	TEST TYPE PERFORMED
☒ Transient	OAE Complete
☐ Distortion Product	☒ OAE Screening
OAE results:	
Right Ear Absent	
Left Ear Absent	

OAE UNIT _____

HEARING AID INFORMATION

RIGHT AID: _____

LEFT AID: _____

OTOSCOPY: _____

HISTORY/IMPRESSIONS/RECOMMENDATIONS: _____

_____

_____

_____

_____

_____

AUDIOLOGIST: _____   ASSISTANT: _____   AUDIOMETER: _____

FIGURE 1.14   Patient 10

PART 1   Audiometric Testing Principles and Audiogram Interpretation

Clinical Enrichment Projects

1. How will the demographics of the U.S. population impact the profession of audiology over the next several decades? In your response address the aging population, cultural and linguistical diversity, and the impact of advances in medical sciences and genetics.

2. Why do you think that gathering case history information is a skill that an audiologist must acquire? Develop your own case history form for either a child, adult, or elderly patient.

3. What are the advantages of insert earphones over super-aural TDH-49 earphones? What is the interaural attenuation value for insert earphones for pure tone and speech audiometry?

4. Discuss the relationship between pure tone and speech audiometric data. How can this information be used to evaluate the impact of hearing loss on an individual's communication abilities?

5. Draw an audiogram that depicts a bilateral, severe, gradually sloping sensorineural hearing loss 250–8000 Hz. Include speech audiometric and immittance data that would be expected based on pure tone thresholds. (See Figure 1.15 for a blank audiogram.)

6. Discuss the relationship between air and bone conduction thresholds for conductive, mixed, and sensorineural hearing loss.

7. Discuss the possible reasons for lack of consistency between pure tone audiometry and speech audiometry.

8. Discuss the relationship between pure tone air and bone conduction audiometry and the results of the immittance battery.

9. Discuss the possible impact of different degrees of hearing loss on communication abilities.

10. What are the advantages of using objective hearing tests such as OAEs and ABR assessments in conjunction with behavioral testing to determine auditory status?

NAME: _____   AGE/DATE OF BIRTH: _____

REFERRED BY: _____   MEDICAL RECORD #: _____

TEST INTERVAL: _____   DATE OF TEST: _____

PURE TONE AUDIOMETRY (RE: ANSI 1996)

HEARING LEVEL IN DECIBELS (dB)

Frequencies: 250, 500, 1000, 2000, 4000, 8000

SPEECH FREQUENCIES: 250, 4000, 8000

KEY:

LEFT	STIMULUS	RIGHT
X	AIR	O
□	AIR - MASK	Δ
>	BONE	<
]	BONE - MASK	[
↘	NO RESPONSE	✓
L	AIDED SOUND FIELD	R
	SOUND FIELD = S	

TEST TYPE
- STANDARD CAE
- PLAY
- COR/VRA
- BOA

TRANSDUCER
- INSERT
- CIRCUMAURAL
- SOUND FIELD

RELIABILITY
- EXCELLENT
- GOOD
- FAIR
- POOR

BOOTH
- #1
- #2 (PEDS)
- #3
- #4 COCH IMPLANT

TYMPANOMETRY (226 Hz)

EAR	LEFT	RIGHT
STATIC ADMITTANCE (mm H_2O)		
TYMP PEAK PRESSURE (DaPa)		
TYMP WIDTH (DaPa)		
EAR CANAL VOLUME cm^3		

LEFT — Admittance — Pressure

RIGHT — Admittance — Pressure

CONTRA	5k Hz	1k Hz	2k Hz	4k Hz	IPSI	.5k Hz	1k Hz	2k Hz	4k Hz
Right (AD) (phone ear)					AD (probe ear)				
Left (AS) (phone ear)					AS (probe ear)				

MIDDLE EAR ANALYZER _____

SPEECH AUDIOMETRY

	PTA	SRT/ SAT	Speech Recognition	Speech Recognition	MCL	UCL
RIGHT (AD)			%	%		
Masking						
LEFT (AS)			%	%		
Masking						

MLV □	CD/tape □	W-22 □	WIPI □	PBK □	SPECIAL:	SPECIAL:
SOUND FIELD			%	%		
RIGHT AIDED			%	%		
LEFT AIDED			%	%		
BINAURAL			%	%		

OTOACOUSTIC EMISSIONS (OAEs)

EMISSION TYPE USED	TEST TYPE PERFORMED
Transient	OAE Complete
Distortion Product	OAE Screening
OAE results:	
Right Ear	
Left Ear	

OAE UNIT _____

HEARING AID INFORMATION

RIGHT AID: _____

LEFT AID: _____

OTOSCOPY: _____

HISTORY/IMPRESSIONS/RECOMMENDATIONS: _____

_____

_____

_____

_____

AUDIOLOGIST: _____   ASSISTANT: _____   AUDIOMETER: _____

FIGURE 1.15 Blank Audiogram

Answers to Audiogram Interpretation Exercises

PATIENT 1

1. *Hearing sensitivity is within normal limits bilaterally.*
2. *The pure tone average in each ear is 12 dB HL.*
3. *Yes, the SRTs in both ears are in good agreement with PTAs because they are within ±5 dB HL of one another.*
4. *The presentation level of the NU#6 words were 40 dB SL re: SRT, which was a presentation level of 50 dB HL in each ear. The word recognition results are excellent bilaterally and suggest no communication problems in quiet when speech is presented at a loud level.*
5. *Tympanograms suggest normal tympanic membrane mobility with normal middle-ear pressure (Type A). Contralateral and ipsilateral acoustic reflexes were within expected levels bilaterally. Acoustic reflex decay was negative at 500 Hz and 1000 Hz bilaterally.*
6. • *Annual audiologic reevaluation to monitor hearing sensitivity due to noise exposure.*
   • *Use of hearing protection when playing the clarinet or exposed to other forms of recreational noise to reduce the likelihood of temporary threshold shift for hearing and tinnitus.*

PATIENT 2

1. *Hearing sensitivity within normal limits at 250–750 Hz with a gradually sloping mild to severe sensorineural hearing loss at 1000–8000 Hz bilaterally.*
2. *The three-frequency pure tone average is 40 dB HL in the right ear and 45 dB HL in the left ear.*
3. *The PTA does not reflect the patient's hearing loss above 2000 Hz, which can impact speech understanding, especially in noise and for high-frequency consonants.*

4. *The interoctave of 750 Hz was tested due to the 20 dB HL difference between 500 Hz and 1000 Hz bilaterally. Testing the interoctave provides more information about the patient's audiometric configuration.*
5. *Normal middle-ear functioning bilaterally.*
6. *Ipsilateral and contralateral acoustic reflexes are within expected levels in each ear based on the patient's degree of hearing loss.*
7. • *Conduct further speech-in-noise testing to gain more information about communication function.*
   • *Administer a hearing handicap scale to determine the self-perception of hearing loss to aid in the development of an audiologic rehabilitation program.*
   • *If a patient reports a communication handicap, recommend hearing aids bilaterally.*
   • *Annual audiologic reevaluation to monitor hearing sensitivity.*

PATIENT 3

1. *The patient exhibits a moderate mixed flat hearing loss at 250–8000 Hz bilaterally.*
2. *Masking was done for bone conduction from 250 Hz, 500 Hz, 1000 Hz, 2000 Hz, and 4000 Hz in both ears due to the 10 dB difference between air conduction and bone conduction thresholds at these frequencies. In order to determine the type of hearing loss, masking was done for bone conductions.*
3. *The thresholds at 2000 Hz in each ear suggest a sensorineural component indicative of Carhart's Notch, which is a classic sign of otosclerosis due to the fixation of the stapes footplate.*

4. Word recognition results were excellent in each ear, which is expected with conductive hearing loss.
5. Tympanograms would suggest stiffness in the middle-ear system due to the presence of otosclerosis (Type A$_s$). Static compliance values would be reduced. Ipsilateral and contralateral reflexes would most likely not be measurable bilaterally due to the conductive pathology in the middle ear.
6. No. OAEs would not be expected due to the presence of conductive pathology in the middle-ear system. In addition, OAEs would not be expected with a hearing loss worse than 35–40 dB HL, which is present in each ear.
7. Otosclerosis.
8. ● Bluish tint to the eyes.
   ● Hearing loss results after pregnancy.
   ● Maternal family history of hearing loss.
   ● Presence of Carhart's Notch at 2000 Hz in each ear.
   ● Shallow tympanograms suggesting stiffness in the middle-ear system.
9. ● Referral to ENT physician for medical consultation.
   ● Trial use of amplification if patient does not want medical and/or surgical intervention at this time.

PATIENT 4

1. Diabetes is a metabolic disease that results from a deficiency of insulin and the inability of the body to use glucose in the normal manner. The potential impact on the auditory mechanism is that the high blood glucose levels can impact the auditory system. Small changes in the blood vessels of the inner ear can compromise blood flow, resulting in sensorineural hearing loss.
2. Hearing sensitivity within normal limits 250–2000 Hz and mild-to-moderate sensorinerual hearing loss 3000–8000 Hz bilaterally.
3. Excellent word recognition ability bilaterally at suprathreshold levels.
4. Yes. There is good agreement between the pure tone averages and SRT in each ear.
5. Normal middle-ear function bilaterally.
6. Otoacoustic emissions are present bilaterally.
7. A 10–15 dB HL shift in hearing thresholds occurred over the last several months. The

patient is exhibiting a moderate-to-severe gradually sloping sensorineural hearing loss 3000–8000 Hz bilaterally. In addition, screening OAEs are not present.
8. Balance testing should be conducted. The dysequilibrium can be the result of a problem within the vestibular system that may not be related to diabetes.
9. ● Continue to monitor hearing sensitivity at least every 3 months until the hearing loss and blood glucose levels stabilize.
   ● Possibly further testing for balance depending on initial balance test results.
   ● Consult with endocronologist about the patient's decrease in hearing sensitivity.

PATIENT 5
Audiogram I

1. Hearing sensitivity is within normal limits bilaterally.
2. Word recognition results were excellent bilaterally.
3. Immittance results suggest normal middle ear function bilaterally.
4. OAEs are present in each ear.

Serial Audiograms 2-4

1. No. The patient's hearing sensitivity has not changed as a result of chemotherapy treatment.
2. Throughout the course of chemotherapy treatments, OAEs should be monitored to determine the impact of treatment on the outer hair cells in the cochlea, which are most sensitivity to ototoxicity.

Audiogram 5

1. A mild-to-moderate sensorineural hearing loss from 4000 Hz to 8000 Hz in each ear that did not exist in previous audiograms.
2. OAEs are absent bilaterally.
3. Damage to the outer hair cells due to ototoxicity from cisplatin treatment.
4. Word recognition scores are excellent bilaterally in quiet despite the presence of a high-frequency hearing loss.
5. No, there are no differences in hearing test results between audiograms 4 and 5; 6 and 7.
6. ● Continue to monitor hearing sensitivity because ototoxic effects can occur up to a year posttreatment.

PATIENT 6

1. *Hearing is within normal limits in the right ear. The hearing sensitivity cannot be determined in the left ear due to inconsistent responses during the test sessions.*
2. • *Presence of OAEs in the left ear despite the reported severity of hearing loss in this ear.*
   • *Presence of contralateral and ipsilateral acoustic reflexes despite the reported severity of the hearing loss in the left ear.*
   • *Excellent word recognition ability when tested at 40 dB SL re: SRT in the left ear. At this suprathreshold level, based on the air conduction thresholds, the patient should not be able obtain a word recognition of 96% with the reported severity of the hearing loss.*
   • *Due to cross-hearing, a shadow curve is present in the left ear.*
3. *The audiometric inconsistencies are probably related to the presence of an exaggerated hearing loss related to the financial compensation for the automobile accident.*
4. *The result of the Speech Stenger is positive, which further helps classify the hearing loss as functional or exaggerated.*
5. *Based on the SRT in the left ear, the patient's hearing sensitivity is most likely within the range of normal hearing.*
6. • *Initiate counseling to resolve the hearing loss.*
   • *Retest after counseling.*
   • *If the functional component is not resolved during the test session, ABR testing should be conducted to estimate hearing threshold levels.*
7. *Financial compensation due to the automobile incident.*

PATIENT 7

1. *Moderately severe 250 Hz–500 Hz rising to moderate 1000 Hz–4000 Hz gradually sloping to severe sensorineural hearing loss bilaterally.*
2. *The pure tone average is 46 dB HL bilaterally.*
3. *Speech recognition scores were 72% in the right ear and 76% in the left ear, which are considered fair in both ears.*
4. *The OAEs are absent bilaterally due to the presence of a moderate hearing loss. There is consistency with the audiogram, as OAEs would not be expected due to the presence of a moderate to moderately severe sensorineural hearing loss.*

5. *Aural fullness, sudden onset hearing loss, tinnitus, and vertigo are consistent with Ménière's disease.*
6. • *Balance testing to determine vestibular function.*
   • *ECOG and possibly ABR.*
7. • *Referral to neuro-otologist.*
   • *Dizziness Handicap Scale; Hearing Handicap Scale.*
   • *Referral to Ménière's support group; possible involvement of spouse.*
   • *Possible amplification once the patient's hearing stabilizes.*
   • *Possible stress management/counseling if patient is depressed and has a reduced quality of life.*

PATIENT 8

1. *The presence of a unilateral sensorineural hearing loss in the left ear. Also of concern is the asymmetrical word recognition scores, the presence of PB-PI rollover, and the lack of acoustic reflexes in the left ear.*
2. *In cases of VIII nerve tumor there is typically a unilateral sensorineural hearing loss. Sometimes, tinnitus is a symptom of a VIII tumor. The presence of rollover is also characteristic of retrocochlear involvement. Contralateral and ipsilateral acoustic reflexes were not measurable in the left ear. These reflexes should be present based on the degree of hearing loss in both ears.*
3. • *ABR.*
   • *Referral back to ENT for neuro-otologic evaluation.*
   • *Vestibular evaluation.*
4. • *Imaging studies.*
5. • *Possible surgical removal of the tumor depending on the size and location.*
   • *No surgical intervention at this time but regular audiologic monitoring of hearing loss in the left ear.*

PATIENT 9

1. *The presence of neurological symptoms including tingling in the extremities, double vision, and dimming of her color perception. In addition, the recent auditory and vestibular symptoms of tinnitus and dizziness are of concern.*

2. *Hearing sensitivity is within normal limits in the left ear. There is a moderate-to-severe sensorineural hearing loss in the right ear.*
3. *Possibly due to retrocochlear or central involvement in the right ear.*
4. *ABR was normal in the left ear and absent in the right ear. The absence of waves I–V suggests neurological involvement.*
5. *Possible etiology is multiple sclerosis, given the patient's age, gender, and neurological symptoms and family history.*

PATIENT 10

1. *Mild-to-moderate gradually sloping sensorineural hearing loss bilaterally 1000 Hz–8000 Hz.*
2. *Word recognition ability is excellent bilaterally.*
3. *The possible etiology of the hearing loss is Ushers II, due to the presence of retinitis pigmentosa and mild to moderate sensorineural hearing loss. Both onsets occurred in adulthood.*
4. *Given the diagnosis of Ushers syndrome, it is recommended that the audiologist work in conjunction with a low-vision specialist to design an appropriate audiologic and visual rehabilitation plan. Ushers II results in progressive loss of vision and hearing; therefore, it is recommended that K. begin counseling to deal with the numerous psychosocial and vocational issues she will face in the future.*

References

American National Standards Institute (ANSI). (1996). *American National Standards specifications for audiometers* (ANSI S 3.6-1996). New York: Author.

American National Standards Institute (ANSI). (1999). *Maximum permissible ambient noise levels for audiometric test rooms.* ANSI 53.1–1999. New York: Author.

American Speech-Language Hearing Association (ASHA). (2003). *Practical forms for audiologists.* Rockville, MD: Author.

American Tinnitus Association. (2007). Retrieved May 10, 2009, from http://www.ata.org

Ballachanda, B. B. (1995). *The human ear canal: Theoretical considerations and clinical applications including cerumen management.* San Diego: Singular.

Battle, D. (2002). *Communication disorders in multicultural population.* Boston: Butterworth Heinemann Boot.

DeBonis, D., & Donohue, C. (2006). *Survey of audiology: Fundamentals for audiologist and health professionals.* Boston: Allyn and Bacon.

Fletcher, H. (1950). A method of calculating hearing loss for speech from an audiogram. *Journal of Acoustical Society of America, 22,* 1–5.

Fletcher, H., & Munson, W. A. (1937). Relation between loudness and masking. *Journal of the Acoustical Society of America, 9,* 1–10.

Hall, J. (2007). *New handbook of auditory evoked responses.* Boston: Allyn and Bacon.

Jerger, J. (1970). Clinical experience with impedance audiometry. *Archives of Otolaryngology, 92,* 311–324.

Jerger, J., Hayes, D. (1976) The cross-check principle in pediatric audiometry. *Archives of Otolaryngology, 102,* 614–620.

Katz, J. (Ed.). (2002). *Handbook of clinical audiology* (5th ed.). Philadelphia: Lippincott Williams & Wilkins.

Kemp, D. T. (1978). Stimulated acoustic emissions from within the human auditory system. *Journal of the Acoustical Society of America, 64,* 1386–1391.

Kochkin, S. (2005). Marko Trak VII. Hearing loss population tops 31 million people. *Hearing Review, 12,* 16–29.

Martin, F. N., Champlin, C. A., & Chambers, J. A. (1998). Seventh survey of audiometric practices in the United States. *Journal of the American Academy of Audiology, 9,* 95–104.

Martin, F. N., & Clark, J. G. (2005). *Introduction to audiology* (9th ed.). Boston: Allyn and Bacon.

Martin, F. N., & Dowdy, L. K. (1986). A modified spondee threshold procedure. *Journal of Auditory Research, 26,* 115–119.

Martin, F. N., & Weller, S. M. (1975). A modified spondee threshold procedure. *Journal of Auditory Research, 26,* 115–229.

Northern, J., & Downs, M. (2002). *Hearing in children* (5th ed.). Philadelphia: Lippincott William & Wilkins.

Stach, B. (1999). *Clinical audiology: An introduction.* San Diego: Singular.

Thorton, A. R., & Raffin, M. J. M. (1978). Speech discrimination scores modified as a binomial variable. *Journal of Speech and Hearing Research,* 21, 507–518.

Trychin, S., & Busacco, D. (1991). *Manual for mental health professionals, Part 1: Basic information for providing services to hard of hearing people and their families.* Washington, DC: Gallaudet University.

Tyler, R. S. (2000). *Tinnitus handbook.* Clifton Park, NY: Thomson Delmar Learning.

U.S. Bureau of the Census. (2000). *Statistical abstract of the United States* (120th ed.). Washington, DC: Author.

Weinstein, B. (2000). *Geriatric audiology.* New York: Thieme.

Yacullo, W. S. (1996). *Clinical masking procedures.* Boston: Allyn and Bacon.

American Academy of Audiology. (2004). Audiology: Scope of practice. *Audiology Today, 16*(3), 44–45.

American Speech-Language-Hearing Association (ASHA). (1978). Guidelines for manual pure-tone audiometry. *Asha, 20,* 297–301.

American Speech-Language-Hearing Association (ASHA). (1990). Guidelines for audiometric symbols. *Asha, 32* (Suppl.), 25–30.

American Speech-Language-Hearing Association (ASHA). (1988). Guidelines for determining the threshold level for speech. *Asha, 30,* 85–89.

Chisolm, T. H., McArdle, R., Abrams, H., & Noe, C. M. (2004). Goals and outcomes of FM used by adults. *The Hearing Journal, 57*(11), 28–35.

Thorton, A. R., & Ruffin, M. J. M. (1978). Speech discrimination scores modeled as a binomial variable. *Journal of Speech and Hearing Research, 21,* 507–518.

Ventry, I., & Weinstein, B. (1982). The Hearing Handicap Inventory for the Elderly. *Ear and Hearing, 3,* 128–133.

Ventry, T. M. (1976). Pure tone-spondee threshold relationship in functional hearing loss. *Journal of Speech & Hearing Disorders, 30,* 377–386.

Audiologic Diagnosis and Management of Hearing Loss in the Pediatric Population

The purpose of this part is to provide an overview of audiological test procedures used with infants, children, and adolescents from birth to 18 years of age. As with other parts in this textbook, it is not meant to be a primary learning tool but rather is a secondary resource to help students analyze and interpret pediatric cases.

STUDENT LEARNING OUTCOMES

On completion of this part students will be able to:

1. Identify guidelines to follow when testing the pediatric population.
2. Identify common hearing disorders found in infants, children, and adolescents.
3. Identify appropriate audiologic testing protocols for the pediatric population based on chronological and developmental ages.
4. Address some of the common concerns in testing infants and children.
5. Interpret audiologic test results for a variety of patients, ages birth to 18 years.
6. Determine the psychological, social, and academic impact of hearing loss on pediatric patients.
7. Provide recommendations for pediatric audiologic rehabilitation.

GENERAL GUIDELINES FOR TESTING THE PEDIATRIC POPULATION

The following are some general guidelines to use in providing services to the pediatric population. These guidelines can help an audiologist be more confident that children with hearing loss will receive the most appropriate audiologic services.

Guideline 1: The audiological assessment techniques selected should be based on the child's developmental age and neuromaturational level rather than chronological age. The ideal testing protocol would include both behavioral and electrophysiological assessments to determine site of lesion and approximate hearing threshold levels between the frequencies of 250 Hz and 4000 Hz. According to Jerger and Hayes (1976), the cross-check principle states that there is no single test result obtained in pediatric assessment that should be considered valid until there is a follow-up test to substantiate the results. If an audiologist bases a diagnostic decision on one behavioral or electrophysiological test, then there could be a misdiagnosis of the hearing loss, which can have devastating long-term consequences on a child's development.

Guideline 2: Audiological testing of the pediatric population should be done over a period of time with ongoing audiological reassessment every six months to one year postdiagnosis until the age of 5 years or until the hearing loss is stable (Northern & Downs, 2002). Genetic counseling should be recommended when a hearing loss of unknown etiology is diagnosed. All family members should receive an audiologic evaluation and genetic counseling in order to determine whether a familial history exists.

Guideline 3: A family-centered approach should be used in the diagnostic and intervention process. The family-centered approach advocates that one or more family members are involved in diagnostic and audiologic rehabilitation management decisions. The family-centered approach is mandated by federal legislation, PL 99-457 and PL 94-142, which involves family members in the development of the Individualized Family Service Plan (IFSP) for children from birth to 3 years of age and the Individualized Education Plan (IEP) for children in preschool through secondary education respectively. Students in secondary education are provided accommodations related to their hearing loss through the Americans with Disabilities Act (ADA).

Guideline 4: Pediatric audiology is a specialization in the profession. A pediatric audiologist needs to have the experience of testing many normal-developing and normal-hearing infants and children in order to gain confidence in diagnosing hearing loss in this population, especially in those children who have a mild-to-moderate hearing loss and are often misdiagnosed or undiagnosed.

Guideline 5: An interdisciplinary team approach should be used in the delivery of hearing health care services. The members of the interdisciplinary team will vary depending on the needs of the child. Interdisciplinary members most likely will include a pediatrician, audiologist, speech-language pathologist, psychologist, teacher or early intervention specialist, social worker, family members, and possibly a pediatric ENT physician.

Guideline 6: The cultural and linguistic diversity of the family must be taken into consideration when providing audiology services. The audiologist and other professionals must be sensitive to the needs of the family and the pace at which the family reaches a level of acceptance of the child's hearing loss. For example, when dealing with a Deaf couple with a deaf child, the family may decide to forgo audiological intervention such as the use of hearing aids or a cochlear implant. Although at times this may be frustrating for the professional, it is in the best interest of the child to respect the family's decisions related to audiologic intervention.

EARLY INFANT HEARING DETECTION PROGRAMS

It has been estimated that approximately 3 in 1,000 babies are born with hearing loss (Northern & Downs, 2002). Over the last several decades, due to improvements in medical technology, many babies with severe medical conditions and disabilities are living longer that in the past. Some of these babies will have a hearing loss that is present at birth or may develop in early childhood. Since 1993, the majority of states have implemented universal hearing screening programs (Joint Committee on Infant Hearing [JCIH], 2007). Such programs conduct a hearing screening using otoacoustic emissions (OAEs) on all well babies and those at risk for hearing loss prior to discharge from the hospital (National Institutes of Health [NIH], 1993). The goal of Early Hearing Detection and Intervention (EDHI) programs is to identify hearing loss at the earliest possible age and provide intervention services such as amplification and/or cochlear implantation. The goal of these programs is to identify hearing loss within the time frame of birth to 3 months of age, with hearing aid fitting done at one month postscreening (JCIH, 2007). The earlier the intervention is initiated, the better the development of speech-language-hearing abilities and literacy skills. It is preferable to identify infants before 3 months of age and offer audiologic intervention before 6 months of age.

An EDHI program offers an OAE screening conducted by a technician who is supervised by an audiologist. The OAE screening of each infant is completed prior to hospital discharge. If the infant fails the OAE screening, then there is a referral for an ABR testing. If the infant fails the ABR, then further behavioral testing should be conducted.

It must be kept in mind that the goal of EDHI is not only to screen infants but also to provide follow-up diagnostic and rehabilitative services. The purpose of a hearing screen is to identify infants with hearing loss and engage in appropriate audiologic management. The follow-up testing will either confirm or negate the presence of hearing loss. The effectiveness of an EDHI program is based upon the number of false-positive and false-negative identification rates. "False positive" in this case refers to referring individuals for follow-up testing after failing the OAE screening when they do not have a hearing loss. "False negative" refers to passing an individual who has a hearing loss. It is better to have a high false-positive referral rate as compared to a high false-negative rate so as not to miss a hearing loss in this population.

Prior to EDHI programs, the average child with hearing loss was identified at 24 to 30 months of age. Identification of children at the age of 24 to 30 months of age will result in possible long-term consequences on speech, language, hearing, cognitive and literacy skills. These children, despite intervention efforts, may not be able to "catch up" to normal developmental milestones (Carney, 1996). If children are not identified at an early age, it may be difficult for them to acquire fundamental literacy skills as well as social skills to achieve success in today's competitive environment, which depends heavily on effective communication skills (e.g., ability to talk on a cell phone, ability to write coherently for email, text messaging skills and basic literacy skills required to function in a "hearing" world).

The consequences of undetected hearing loss include impact on speech-language skills and literacy skills. There also may be potential effects on academic achievement, social development, and family dynamics. Despite early identification programs, there is still a lag in providing intervention services such as hearing aid fitting, cochlear implantation, auditory training, and speech-language intervention (Northern & Downs, 2002). There are a variety of reasons for this, including parental denial of hearing loss, parents being overwhelmed with their new role, lack of knowledge about follow-up audiologic services, lack of transportation to services, lack of medical insurance, and cultural differences related to acceptance of and intervention for a hearing loss. Audiologic intervention needs to be consistent with the Individuals with Disabilities Education Act (IDEA) in that a family-centered intervention approach is advocated. Public Law 102-119 and PL 94-142 provide the guidelines for developing and implementing Individualized Family Service Plans (IFSP). The Federal Education of the Handicapped Act (PL 102-119) provides for statewide comprehensive, coordinated, interdisciplinary, and interagency programs of early intervention services for all children with disabilities and their families in order to meet the developmental needs of each child.

Another goal of an EDHI program is to reduce the cost of associated with special education services and to produce adults who can enter the work force and be productive members of society. It has been estimated that the $79 billion spent per year associated with hearing loss may be reduced by 3.9 billion per year or more as a result of neonatal detection and early intervention (Northern & Downs, 2002). As the economy inflation rate increases, so will the cost of special education services. The major task for hospital administrators is to weigh the cost and benefits associated with universal hearing screening programs and decide whether the costs outweigh the risks associated with early detection of hearing loss. However, the fact that EDHI programs are mandated by state legislation makes hospitals comply with this valuable program. It is imperative that audiologists make the results of EDHI known to the hospital administrators and state legislators on a consistent basis so that these services will be funded.

PEDIATRIC AUDIOLOGIC ASSESSMENT

The pediatric audiologic assessment should make use of tests that have the same goal as those used with adults; however, the test procedures must be modified to take into account the development and chronological age of the child. The results obtained from the pediatric hearing test should result in the same outcomes as those from an adult evaluation; that is, to determine the type and degree of hearing loss so that auditory rehabilitation intervention can be implemented as early as possible. If the initial audiologic testing results suggest a hearing loss but the degree is not definitive, the audiologist can initiate auditory rehabilitation and continue to modify the intervention plan until more definitive results about the hearing loss are obtained.

Case History Interview

The audiologic diagnostic evaluation of the pediatric population should begin with an extensive case history interview. The case history for children is typically longer than the case history for adults and elderly patients. It may be helpful for parents to fill out the case history form in advance of the child's appointment so that they can refer to their pediatric medical records. It is recommended that the audiologist should review the pertinent information with a parent or primary caregiver at the time of the evaluation. The case history should include information related to prenatal, perinatal, and postnatal histories. Prenatal history would include information on the progression of pregnancy and any complications that arose. Perinatal history includes any problems during labor and delivery of the infant. Postnatal history would include any complications that occurred after delivery, medical problems, child's developmental history and milestone achievement, concerns parents or other family members have about the child's hearing and/or speech and language, presence of other disabilities, educational history, and any other areas that provide information to help the audiologist in the diagnosis of the hearing loss and the determination of the possible etiology. Refer to the sample pediatric case history provided by the American Speech-Language-Hearing Association (2003) in Figure 2.1.

The audiologist should review the case history information during the initial phase of the diagnostic testing. Each clinic should adapt a pediatric case history form dependent on the population for whom the clinical services are provided. For example, if the clinic sees a large number of premature infants, then that section of the case history form should be expanded so as to capture critical information. The case history should be flexible in content to meet the needs of the clinical population being served. This information is a critical part of the audiological evaluation and can assist the audiologist in determining the possible etiology of the hearing loss. In addition, the audiologist should query the parents about other professional services that the child has received so that the results of the audiologic evaluation can be sent to these professionals in case an interdisciplinary treatment plan is required.

Behavioral Testing of Children

The following is a brief summary of the behavioral test procedures used with the pediatric population. For more information on pediatric audiology testing, refer to the References and Recommended Readings at the end of this part. Despite the advent of electrophysiological measures, it is critical for the audiologist to engage in behavioral testing to observe the physiological responses of the young child to auditory stimuli. In order to obtain information about each ear, the

Pediatric Audiologic Assessment

Practitioner Name or Practice
Address
City, State Zipcode
Phone Number - Fax Number
Web site - E-mail Address

Child Case History

Name: Date:

1. For what reason was this hearing test arranged?

2. Has your child ever had a hearing test?   ☐ Yes ☐ No

3. Do you have any concerns about your child's hearing?   ☐ Yes ☐ No

4. Does your child seem to hear better on some days than other? ☐ Yes ☐ No

5. Does anyone in the family (sisters, brothers, aunts, grandparents, etc.)
   have a handicap or problem with language, learning, hearing, speech, etc.?
                                                              ☐ Yes ☐ No

6. Were there any complications during pregnancy or delivery? ☐ Yes ☐ No

7. Were any of the following present after your child's birth or during the first two
   months?

   ☐ Stayed in hospital after mother   ☐ Prematurity

   ☐ Birth weight less than 5 lbs.   ☐ Poor weight gain

   ☐ Did not respond to sounds or people   ☐ Appeared yellow

   ☐ Was in an incubator or isolette   ☐ Infections at birth

   ☐ Difficulty breathing   ☐ Physical deformities

   ☐ High fever

8. What is your child's general health?   ☐ Good ☐ Average ☐ Poor

FIGURE 2.1 ASHA Sample Pediatric Case History

American Speech-Language-Hearing Association (ASHA) (2003). *Practical forms for audiologists* Rockwille, MD.

PART 2 Audiologic Diagnosis and Management of Hearing Loss in the Pediatric Patient

9. Is your child taking any medication now? ☐ Yes ☐ No

10. Has your child ever been hospitalized? ☐ Yes ☐ No

11. Has your child experienced ear infections or other ear disorders? ☐ Yes ☐ No

12. Has your child had any ear surgery? ☐ Yes ☐ No

13. What illnesses has your child had?

☐ High fever	☐ Dizziness
☐ Convulsions	☐ Pneumonia
☐ Measles	☐ Heart problems
☐ Head or ear injury	☐ Rheumatic fever
☐ Encephalitis	☐ Allergies
☐ Meningitis	☐ Asthma
☐ Tonsillitis	☐ Other: _____

14. Has your child ever received speech therapy? ☐ Yes ☐ No

15. Do you have any concerns about your child's speech and language? ☐ Yes ☐ No

16. Do you have any concerns about your child's physical or mental development? ☐ Yes ☐ No

17. If your child attends school, has he or she repeated any grades? ☐ Yes ☐ No

18. Do you believe your child has any learning problems? ☐ Yes ☐ No

19. What questions would you like to have answered as a result of today's hearing test?

_____

FIGURE 2.1 *(Continued)*

audiologist should use insert earphones. Insert earphones will prevent collapsed ear canals in this population, and more important, will yield information about hearing sensitivity in each ear. Bone conduction testing also should be done on young children to determine the type of hearing loss. A major caution for audiologists who conduct behavioral testing is the possible influence of tester bias in determining whether a behavioral response was present. One way to prevent tester bias is to have several individuals assess whether the child has responded to the test stimuli. The typical arrangement with young children is for one audiologist to conduct the testing on the examiner's side of the test suite and the other audiologist to be with the young patient to assist with the conditioning of the child. In addition, testing the young child over several sessions may provide more data on the reliability and the validity of the behavioral responses over time and across test sessions. It should be the primary goal of the audiologist to gather behavioral and objective test results to estimate hearing threshold levels as early as possible so that audiologic intervention can be initiated.

Behavioral Observation Audiometry

Behavioral observation audiometry (BOA) is used to assess infants from birth to about 6 months of age. BOA involves the audiologist's observing the infant's behavior in response to sound. Audiologists need to be astute observers of the infant's behavior to auditory stimuli. Some of the infant's responses to sound may include eye blinking, eye widening, increase or cessation of sucking, increase or cessation of crying, and searching for sound. It is important to realize that the information obtained from pediatric test such as BOA should be classified as the child's minimum levels of response (MLRs) because it is not certain that the responses represent the lowest intensity level that the infant or young child can hear (Matkin & Wilcox, 1999). As part of BOA testing, the audiologist should present a loud stimulus greater than 65 dB HL to assess whether the Moro Reflex is present. This reflex will be absent if a moderately severe or greater hearing loss exists and can help the audiologist in the diagnostic process.

Visual Reinforcement Audiometry

Visual reinforcement audiometry (VRA) can be used with children from about 6 months of age, possibly younger, through about 18 months to 2 years of age. The goal of VRA testing is to observe the child responsing to auditory stimuli by turning to the source of the sound emanating from a loudspeaker or earphones. The initial phase of testing involves conditioning the child to turn toward a visual stimulus such as a lighted animal in Plexiglas as a response to auditory stimuli. In addition, more current VRA techniques use video-recorded stimuli. The audiologist must observe that the child's response is time-locked to the presentation of the stimulus. One problem associated with VRA is the habituation of the behavioral response, which can cause the test result to lack reliability and validity. *Habituation* refers to the decrease in the infant's response to auditory stimuli over time due to boredom with the task (Northern & Downs, 2002). One way to deal with habituation is by changing the reinforcement for the child on a regular basis during the test session so as to hold the child's attention. Once the audiologist obtains a consistent response from the child, it is best to reduce the reinforcement to an intermittent basis. Intermittent reinforcement should keep the child's attention; thereby reducing the habituation of the behavioral response and allowing for more responses to be obtained. Children with visual and/or motor problems may not be able to participate in the VRA task, and depending on the chronological and developmental age, one or more other behavioral tests may be recommended.

Conditioned Orientation Reflex Audiometry   Conditioned orientation reflex (COR) is a higher-level conditioning task than VRA. COR is applicable for children 24 to 36 months of age. For COR, the task is to have the child orient or turn to the location of the acoustic stimulus. For example, if the acoustic stimulus is presented through the left earphone or left soundfield speaker, the child's task is to turn to that side and, on successfully doing so, receive the visual reinforcer presented on the same side as the acoustic stimulus. COR provides important information about a child's localization ability.

Conditioned Play Audiometry   Conditioned play audiometry can be used effectively with children aged 36 months to 5 years. Most normally developing children can engage in play audiometry beginning at age 3. Play audiometry involves conditioning the child to respond to an auditory stimulus via a play technique, such as dropping a block in a can or placing a peg in a board. The play activity can vary depending on the age and interest level of the child. One advantage of play audiometry is that the play task can be changed frequently once the child is conditioned so as to avoid habituation of the response. Conditioned play audiometry can be used for pure tone and speech testing. The child will need to be reconditioned for speech testing because it requires a different task than does pure tone testing. Play audiometry can be useful technique with persons who have developmental challenges such as mental retardation or autism. The type of pediatric test protocol chosen will depend on the developmental and chronological age of the child and his or her motivation to perform the task, attention, and interest levels. The pediatric audiologist must be astute in evaluating the child using the most appropriate test protocol(s) so that accurate, reliable, and valid test results are obtained and the most appropriate age-related audiologic intervention strategies can be initiated (see Table 2.1).

TABLE 2.1   Age-Appropriate Behavioral Tests: Chronological Age and Associated Behavioral Test in Children

Age	Behavioral Test
Birth–6 months	BOA
6–24 months	VRA & COR Audiometry
24–36 months	COR Audiometry
3–5 years	Play Audiometry
5 years and older	Conventional Audiometry

Pediatric Audiologic Assessment

Speech Audiometry Testing in Children

There are a variety of speech tests that can be done to determine a child's ability to understand speech under different listening conditions. As mentioned previously, the type of speech test selected will depend on the chronological and developmental age of the child. Many audiologists prefer to start the audiology test with speech testing followed by pure tones. The reasons for this are that the speech stimulus is more interesting to the child than pure tones and is composed of a complex frequency spectrum, thereby giving more information about hearing status. The results of the speech testing can serve as a benchmark to indicate the reliability of responses to pure tones. Speech testing also can be done via bone conduction to assess whether a conductive pathology is present. Speech testing provides a great deal of information regarding communication abilities of the child under a variety of listening situations. The following sections review some of the more commonly used speech assessments for the pediatric population.

Speech detection/speech awareness threshold in children. In young children, it may not be possible to attain a speech reception threshold (SRT). In such cases, the speech detection threshold or speech awareness threshold (SDT/SAT) should be obtained. It should be noted that the SDT/SAT has limited diagnostic value. It can be used to estimate the SRT; however, the SDT/SAT is usually 10–15 dB HL lower, or better, than the SRT. The SDT/SAT cannot be used to predict the pure tone thresholds in the speech range, especially in the case of high-frequency hearing loss. The pure tone thresholds, however, can be used to predict the SDT/SAT in some cases such as in flat audiograms. The SDT/SAT should never be used as the "only" test in the diagnosis of childhood hearing loss because erroneous results can result. Most often, the SDT/SAT is obtained using stimuli such as the child's name, continuous discourse, CV syllabi, or short phrases. In order to obtain accurate results, it is critical to use speech stimuli so that the child can understand as well as pay attention during the test session.

Speech reception threshold testing in children. For children 4 years of age or older, a speech reception threshold (SRT) may be obtained using the CID W-1 children's spondee list. Children with expressive or receptive speech and language deficits can provide a nonverbal response such as pointing to spondee picture cards or pointing to objects representing the spondee words (e.g., airplane, baseball, toothbrush). The SRT can be useful in gaining information about the child's hearing sensitivity in the frequency region of 500–2000 Hz, but overall has limited diagnostic value by itself.

Word recognition testing in children. The results of the word recognition testing can provide information to help the audiologist understand the impact of the hearing loss on the speech-understanding abilities of the child, especially at loud levels in quiet. This information is critical to help determine the type and severity of hearing loss and to obtain valuable information for audiologic rehabilitation recommendations (e.g., hearing aids, assistive listening devices, and/or cochlear implants). The Phonetically Balanced Kindergarten (PB-K) word lists are appropriate for children as young as 4 years of age and as old as 5½ years of age who can provide a verbal response. Children 5½ years of age and older who are normally developing should be tested using either the NU#6 or CID W-22 word list. It is recommended that audiologists use live-voice testing instead of recorded materials to keep the child's attention. The interpretation of the word recognition score for children is the same as for adults, with a maximum score of 100% and a lowest score of 0%. Word recognition test results can be very valuable in determining the most appropriate audiologic intervention such as determining the possible benefit from amplification devices.

In testing children under 5 years of age, there are a variety of additional speech tests that can be used to assess speech understanding. Some of the more commonly used speech assessments for this population include the following:

Northwestern University Children with Hearing Impairment (NU-CHIPS) (Elliot & Katz, 1980)—This closed-response task comprises 50 monosyllabic words selected based on the vocabulary level of normally developing children aged 2½ years and older. It is composed of 65 word pictures, with 6 pictures per foil. This test is very useful for children with hearing loss who also may have speech and language deficits.

Word Intelligibility by Picture Identification (WIPI) (Ross & Lerman, 1970)—WIPI is a six-item closed-response picture identification task that is appropriate for children 5 years of age and older. The child is asked to point to the picture of the word presented. It is recommended that the audiologist use the incorrect word responses to analyze a child's auditory confusions. Such information may be helpful for purposes of speech perception training.

Monosyllabic-Trochee-Spondee Test (MST) (Erber, 1982)—This word recognition test uses a closed-set format with 12 words comprising of monosyllabic, trochees, and spondee words. The test is designed to identify stress patterns. It is most useful for children who are deaf or cochlear implantees.

Objective Testing of the Pediatric Population

The best approach in working with the pediatric population is to use a combination of behavioral (i.e., subjective) and objective (e.g., electrophysiological) tests. By combining these two types of evaluation tools, the audiologist can be more certain in diagnosing the hearing loss in infants and young children or those who are mentally challenged. Objective tests that provide valuable information about the physiological integrity of the auditory system include immittance, OAEs, and auditory evoked potentials. These tests tend to be cost-effective with high sensitivity and specificity to determine hearing loss in pediatric patients.

TABLE 2.2 Age-Appropriate Speech Tests and Materials: Speech Assessment and Stimuli in Children Birth–5 Years of Age

Test	Speech Stimuli	Population
SDT/SAT	Running Speech	Infants–3 years
SRT	Children's Spondees	3–4 years
Speech Recognition	PB-K WIPI NU-CHIPS MST	4–5 years

Immittance testing in children. Immittance testing is very important for children due to the high incidence of conductive hearing loss primarily from otitis media. One of the major problems in conducting immittance testing in infants and young children is the influence of movements and muscle artifacts that can contaminate the results. During tympanometry and acoustic reflex measurements children need to remain very still. This is often a challenging task because these tests tend to be frightening for children. It is best to conduct immittance testing when the child is calm and possibly sleeping so as to eliminate muscle artifacts. When testing children who are awake, the audiologist or the parent should distract the child using toys or videos to promote stillness during the evaluation.

Oftentimes, when testing young children, it is difficult to obtain the complete immittance test battery. The audiologist may be able to obtain only a tympanogram and ipsilateral acoustic reflex screening in each ear. Acoustic reflex testing is usually not done in this population because of the amount of time required and the difficulty of keeping many young children still during this test. It is critical that, when a child has pressure equalization (P.E.) tubes, the audiologist measure the volume of the middle-ear cavity to determine whether the P.E. tubes are patent. When the P.E. tubes are patent, there will be a large volume measurement for the middle-ear system. It is recommended that pediatricians or their staff also conduct tympanometry when a middle-ear infection is suspected so as to monitor the progression and recovery of otitis media during and after medical treatment. In cases of significant negative middle-ear pressure less than or equal to 150 daPa, it may be best to monitor the child using tympanometry at 6- to 8-week intervals to assess whether either the negative middle-ear pressure has resolved or if there has been progression to otitis media with the presence of infectious or noninfectious fluid.

McCandless and Alfred (1978) reported that, with a 220 Hz probe tone, only 4% of 53 infants younger than 48 hours demonstrated acoustic reflexes. When the probe tone frequency was increased to 660 Hz, 89% of the same infant subjects demonstrated acoustic reflexes. These researchers concluded that, when doing immittance testing on infant, a 660 Hz tone should be used to elicit acoustic reflexes. Bennett (1984) found that the optimal frequency for eliciting the acoustic reflexes in neonates is about 1400 Hz; however, most audiologists continue using either a 220 Hz or 660 Hz probe tone, which may lead to misdiagnosis of the acoustic reflex data. For older children, the audiologist should be able to obtain the complete immittance battery including tympanometry, static acoustic compliance, and acoustic reflex measurements. Acoustic reflex decay testing is usually not conducted in infants and children unless there is some genetic and/or medical condition that may cause VII and/or VIII nerve damage or damage to the brainstem (e.g., tumors, Fetal Alcohol Syndrome, neurofibromatosis Type I and Type II). Refer to Northern and Downs (2002) for a complete description of medical and genetic conditions with associated hearing disorders in childhood.

The information obtained from the immittance battery can be useful in determining the site of lesion and estimation of hearing threshold levels. This data will augment behavioral results and also will provide objective information about the integrity of the middle-ear system. Immittance results used in conjunction with behavioral testing and other electrophysiological measurements, such as OAEs and ABR, can provide the audiologist with extensive information to aid in the diagnosis of the hearing loss so that early intervention can be initiated.

Otoacoustic emissions testing in children.   Otoacoustic emissions (OAEs) testing is very useful in evaluating the status of outer hair cell functioning in the cochlea in infants and young children. It is a quick and reliable screening tool. OAEs will be present in normal hearing and mild sensorineural hearing loss. OAEs will not be present if a hearing loss is greater than 30–35 dB HL or possibly in the presence of a conductive hearing loss (Kemp, 1978). For cost effectiveness, it is recommended that if OAEs are absent at the time of screening then immittance testing should be done prior to discharge from the hospital. Gathering additional information about the middle-ear system may eliminate the number of false-positive referrals for follow-up audiologic testing that may be related to debris in the ear canal or fluid in the middle ear. In cases of premature or ill infants, OAEs can be especially useful in monitoring the effects of ototoxic medications, especially those used to keep the neonate alive, such as mycin drugs (Campbell, 2006). Fortunately, OAEs usually can be obtained within the first several hours after birth and are not dependent on the maturation of the auditory system. Therefore, they can provide good diagnostic information especially when used in conjunction with other audiologic tests.

OAEs can be very useful in evaluating the presence of functional or nonorganic hearing loss and are more cost-effective than an ABR assessment for the pediatric population. If the OAEs are normal, then the audiologist can suggest additional tests that can determine whether there is a functional hearing loss in a young child or adolescent. Distortion-product otoacoustic emissions (DPOAEs) are tonal responses located at frequencies determined by two simultaneously presented pure tones with frequencies F_1 and F_2. The results are DPOAEs at various distortion product frequencies (Hayes & Northern, 1990). DPOAEs should be done on pediatric patients if hearing loss is suspected.

Auditory brainstem response testing in children.   Auditory brainstem response (ABR) can be a very useful tool in evaluating children for whom reliable behavioral results cannot be obtained. The latency-intensity function for wave V can provide

Pediatric Audiologic Assessment

information on the type of hearing loss and approximate hearing threshold level. In children younger than 18 months of age, the ABR is different morphologically than for older children and adults. The ABR for very young children is typically characterized by the presence of waves I and V with all other waves being absent (Hall, 2007). The amplitude of the response is reduced in young children. The absolute and interpeak latencies of waves are increased but move more toward the norms for adults as the child matures. Typically, there are separate norms established for infants younger than 18 months of age for each clinical site. In children who are very uncooperative, it may be necessary to sedate the child for the ABR testing. Sedation does not influence the ABR, and in most cases the child will remain asleep during the test session.

The goal in working with young children is to obtain as much information as possible from the ABR in a short amount of time while the child is quiet or under sedation. In the past, a screening ABR was used to test infants and young children. However, given the amount of information that can be obtained about the type and degree of hearing loss, it is recommended that a diagnostic ABR be performed whenever possible rather than using an ABR screening tool if hearing loss is suspected.

Another advantage of ABR is that bone conduction thresholds can be obtained to gain information about the integrity of the sensorineural mechanism. The results should be consistent with latencies typically found for air conduction ABR. One of the major limitations is the maximum power output level of the bone conduction oscillator, especially for low-frequency stimuli. The best type of acoustic stimuli to use for ABR bone conduction testing is tone pips (Hall, 2007).

SPECIAL CONSIDERATIONS IN THE PEDIATRIC POPULATION

The following are some special issues and considerations that apply primarily to audiological evaluation of children with hearing loss.

Masking in Children

Whenever a hearing loss is present, masking may be necessary in order to obtain true auditory thresholds. Masking should be attempted in testing children as often as possible. Some children will not be able to differentiate between the masking noise and the test stimuli, whereas other children may respond only to loud test stimuli. One of the advantages of insert earphones is that, because of the high interaural attenuation values, possibly as much as 50–70 dB HL, there may not be a need to mask for air conduction testing. When given appropriate instructions, most young children can participate in a masking task so as to determine the type of hearing loss.

Otitis Media in Children

Otitis media is an inflammation of the middle ear and is characterized by the presence of negative middle-ear pressure and possible fluid, which is known as otitis media with effusion. Stach (1999) reported that more than 29 types of otitis media exist. The total medical cost related to otitis media in the United States is estimated to be $5 billion per year (Northern & Downs, 2002). Otitis media is the number one reason for childrens' visits to a pediatrician in the Unites States. Nearly 30 million visits to pediatricians occur per year related to the diagnosis and treatment of otitis media. These visits include emergency room costs, follow-up with the pediatrician, and medical costs associated with an ENT physician evaluation, audiologic and speech-language-pathology evaluations, and interventions. Before the age of 6 years, approximately 85% to 90% of children will have at least one bout of otitis media. Nearly 20% of children with recurrent otitis media will require the placement of P.E. tubes (Northern & Downs, 2002).

In some children, a hearing loss will accompany otitis media. It may range from slight to moderate in degree. The underlying cause of otitis media is related to Eustachian tube dysfunction, which leads to the production of fluid by the mucosal lining of the middle ear. Otitis media is a common condition in children due to the Eustachian tube being more horizontal, shorter, and composed of more-flaccid cartilage compared to that of adults (Stach, 1999). Typically, the Eustachian tube is developed by age 7 or 8 years, which results in a decrease in the number of episodes of otitis media; however, there will be a small group of children for whom otitis media will be a chronic condition and may continue into adulthood. In this subpopulation, it is critical to determine the underlying cause of otitis media because it may be related to allergies or some other underlying medical condition (e.g., upper respiratory infections) (Northern & Downs, 2002).

There are some risk factors related to otitis media. Children are at higher risk if parents and siblings have histories of otitis media. Children from low socioeconomic environments are at higher risk, as they may not have access to health care. Children exposed to secondary cigarette smoke or who attend day care also may be at higher risk for otitis media. Children with Down's syndrome and craniofacial anomalies tend to be at higher risk for otitis media than the general population due to the high incidence of upper respiratory infections (Northern & Downs, 2002).

Children with chronic otitis media that does not resolve need to be followed by an audiologist for months or perhaps years. It is necessary to follow these children to ascertain whether they have conductive hearing loss and/or other complications such as cholesteatoma or perforated tympanic membrane. It also is not known at this time whether there are any long-term effects from numerous bouts of otitis media, such as speech and language development and/or auditory processing disorders (APD). Children with chronic otitis media may benefit from the use of a mild-gain FM system in the classroom or a bone-anchored hearing aid (BAHA) depending on the frequency of the bouts of otitis media and the impact on academic and social achievement.

Unilateral Hearing Loss in Children

Twenty-five out of every 1,000 children in the Unites States will have a significant hearing loss that interferes with learning and education (Bess, 1985). Of these children, two-thirds have a unilateral sensorineural hearing loss that results in deficits of sound localization and speech recognition especially in difficult listening environments such as noise and (Bess & Tharpe, 1984). These authors reported that children with unilateral hearing loss exhibit educational and/or behavioral problems in school. Bess and Tharpe (1984) stated that children with unilateral hearing loss are more prone to academic difficulties as compared to normal-hearing children. They found that in a study of 60 children with unilateral hearing loss nearly 50% experienced academic failure and required special assistance such as learning resources. Many children with unilateral hearing loss may benefit from the use of a hearing aid and/or assistive listening device to improve their overall communication functioning, especially in the classroom and other noisy environments. These children also should engage in communication strategies training so that appropriate strategies can be used when a communication breakdown occurs or to prevent such breakdowns.

Auditory Processing Disorders in Children

There are some children who do not have a peripheral hearing loss, but exhibit deficits in processing auditory stimuli. Central auditory processing disorders (CAPD) refer to problems with the processing of auditory information with problems noted in the following skills: sound localization, sound lateralization, auditory discrimination, auditory pattern recognition, temporal processing, and performance with degraded acoustic signals (ASHA, 2005). The referenced term today is *auditory processing disorder* (APD) but is used interchangeably with *CAPD*.

Information processing involves perceptual, cognitive, and linguistic skills that result in effective receptive communication of auditory stimuli. According to ASHA (1993), an *auditory processing disorder* refers to limitations in the ongoing transmission, analysis, organization, transformation, storage, retrieval, and use of information in the audible signal.

Testing for auditory processing disorders in children under 7 years of age is controversial (Katz, 2002). Some audiologists believe that many of the existing central auditory processing tests are difficult for children to do and therefore believe they lack reliability and validity. In the References and Recommendation Readings sections of this textbook, there are resources that will provide more information about tests to assess auditory processing abilities in children.

Attention-Deficit/Hyperactivity Disorder and Auditory Processing Disorder

The relationship between attention-deficit/hyperactivity disorder (ADHD) and APD is not clear. Chermak, Hall, and Musiek (1999) stated that ADHD tends to be associated with more global disruption of sensory information, whereas APD is the result of problems with auditory processing. Not all children with ADHD exhibit auditory processing problems. However, there may be a correlation between ADHD and APD, and further investigation is warranted.

Auditory Neuropathy in Children

A very rare condition that young children may exhibit is auditory neuropathy. Sininger, Hood, Starr, Berlin, and Picton (1995) stated that some of the audiological characteristics for auditory neuropathy include a sensorineural hearing loss that can range from mild to profound and may fluctuate, normal OAEs, absent or severely abnormal ABR, and absent acoustic ipsilateral and contralateral acoustic reflexes. Auditory neuropathy is believed to be a function of a lesion(s) central to the cochlea and may be the result of lack of neuron firing (Sininger et al., 1995). Oftentimes, this disorder is treated in the same manner as a sensorineural hearing loss using amplification. There is a fair amount of success with hearing aids. Some infants and children with this disorder have undergone cochlear implant surgery with some success. Typically, it will be very difficult for a child with auditory neuropathy to learn language solely through audition. This child may benefit from learning sign language or cued speech in conjunction with other rehabilitation techniques (Northern & Downs, 2002).

Functional Hearing Loss in Children

There will be a small population of children who exhibit a functional hearing loss. In most cases, the child may be experiencing some type of traumatic situation or change in lifestyle. The functional hearing loss will provide the child with attention or an excuse for inappropriate behaviors or actions. Some children who are having academic or social problems may feign a hearing loss. Another instance that is often seen is when parents are going through a divorce and their child may pretend to have a hearing loss for psychological reasons related to family issues. Children usually are not savvy when it comes to exhibiting behaviors that are consistent with a functional hearing loss. If the audiologist thinks the child is exhibiting a functional hearing loss, then it is best to start the testing with objective assessments such as otoacoustic emissions (OAEs) and immittance testing. The information obtained from these tests will provide information about the integrity of the auditory system and possible degree of hearing loss. In any case, the audiologist should refer the child and family for psychological counseling even if the hearing loss is resolved, because it is abnormal for a child to exhibit a functional hearing loss. In addition, it is not certain whether the child's behaviors will resolve without some type of psychological intervention. The school should be notified about this abnormal response because the child may continue to exhibit behaviors consistent with hearing loss, especially if academic difficulties are present.

Children with Physical and/or Mental Challenges

Oftentimes, children with physical and/or mental challenges are difficult to test and may need modifications to the pediatric test battery. For example, when assessing difficult-to-test populations, there may be a greater reliance on objective assessments instead of subjective audiometric procedures. Children who are considered to be challenging to test may need to be seen over several test sessions in order to establish reliable and consistent responses to auditory stimuli. Some of the common problem areas in testing children with physical and/or mental challenges are reduced attention span and problems adjusting to the test environment, leading to inconsistent responses. The test protocol will need to be adjusted depending on the child's unique needs. For example, a child with visual impairments or poor head and neck control may not be able to engage in VRA or COR testing. One of the most challenging populations to test is children who have been identified as autistic. These children may not respond to any auditory stimuli or may be hypersensitive to auditory stimuli due to sensory integration problems. It may be necessary to sedate such a child to obtain ABR thresholds, OAEs, and immittance results. Hopefully, over time, behavioral thresholds can be obtained to substantiate the electrophysiological responses. The clinical pediatric audiologist needs to be creative in trying to elicit consistent behavioral responses from the child with physical and/or mental challenges. It is critical that the pediatric audiologist be aware of the developmental age of the child so as to use tests that are appropriate based on the child's mental and developmental age as compared to chronological age. Today, due to the numerous objective tests, good diagnostic information can be obtained so that audiologic intervention can be started to facilitate speech-language development and facilitate literacy skills and academic performance.

INTERVENTION WITH FAMILIES FROM CULTURALLY AND LINGUISTICALLY DIVERSE BACKGROUNDS

As the United States population becomes more culturally and linguistically diverse, it is critical that audiologists be aware of some of the unique characteristics of helping families from various racial and ethnic groups. Most audiologists will not be able to become familiar with all characteristics of every culturally and linguistically diverse group; however, some general areas should be investigated when dealing with families of children who are diagnosed as deaf or hard-of-hearing.

One area that the audiologist should investigate in advance of the first meeting with the family is how its particular culture typically views a child's disability. In some cultures a disability such as hearing loss is viewed as a "Godsend." In other cultures, families view the child's disability as "shame" and related to some wrongdoing on the part of the parents in the past. This information is critical to know, as it will have profound implications for auditory rehabilitation. If parents perceive the disability as a result of some wrongdoing, then they may not be interested in participating in the rehabilitation process. As much as this is to the detriment to the child, the family wishes must be acknowledged. For some families, counseling with a professional from their cultural/linguistic background may help the family accept the child's hearing loss (Battle, 2002).

AUDIOLOGIC INTERVENTION FOR CHILDREN WITH HEARING LOSS

There are a variety of audiologic intervention techniques that can be used effectively with the pediatric population. This textbook is not designed to address audiologic management techniques for children; however, general information will be presented in this section.

Amplification Devices for Children

The majority of children with hearing loss will use hearing aids and hopefully assistive listening devices such as an FM system. The type of amplification recommended is based on the degree of hearing loss, type of hearing loss, and age of the child. For most children, it is best to recommend behind-the-ear (BTE) digital programmable hearing aids. Behind-the-ear hearing aids are preferred over in-the-ear hearing aids because it is not as costly to replace the earmold, direct audio input is available for most BTE aids, and stronger t-coils are the norm. Children should use a combination of hearing aids and assistive listening devices as much as possible so as to improve the signal-to-noise ratio and improve speech understanding ability, especially in group situations, background noise reverberation, and large areas. As soon as a child's hearing loss is diagnosed, amplification should be fit and other types of audiologic rehabilitation implemented (e.g., auditory training, auditory-visual integration training, and communication strategies training). It is critical that children's amplification devices are cared for and maintained on a regular basis. Annual audiologic reevaluation and hearing aid checks also are necessary to ensure the child's amplification devices are working properly.

Cochlear Implants for Children

Research is being conducted to investigate the optimum age for cochlear implantation in infants and young children (Holt & Svirsky, 2008). In the past decade, cochlear implantation was restricted by the Food and Drug Administration (FDA) to children 2 years of age and older. Since the mid 2000s, cochlear implants are being done as early as 6 months of age. Current research is being conducted to investigate how infants with cochlear implants perceive and develop speech and language (Tyler, 2006). One question that arises is whether there are significant differences in development of speech and language in children implanted at 6 months of age as compared to 1 year of age. Current literature indicates that the brain begins to solidify its development of speech and language before age 3. This research suggests that children who are implanted at an earlier age may develop speech and language in a manner similar to normal-hearing children. It appears that infants who have been implanted at about 6 months of age may need some time to adjust to the cochlear implant in order for the brain to interpret speech and language to the same extent as a hearing infant. In addition, research suggests that there are significant advantages in bilateral cochlear implantation in the pediatric population (Galvin, Mok, Dowel, & Briggs, 2008).

Educational Options for Children

The majority of children with hearing loss who are hard of hearing usually are educated in the regular classroom (Northern & Downs, 2002). Children who are hard of hearing are the most underserved of all children with disabilities. Often-times, the hearing loss is not identified and the child struggles in the regular classroom without the appropriate learning and emotional support services. These children tend to experience problems socially and emotionally. There are a variety of educational options available for children with hearing loss. The choice of educational setting is dependent on a number of factors including age of onset of hearing loss, ability to communicate, literacy level, preference of the family, and logistical issues such as geographical location and availability of the services. The type of educational setting will be determined by a number of vari-ables including communication abilities and style, cognitive, social, and famil-ial preference. It is vital that each school system engage the services of educational audiologists in order to better ensure the most appropriate services are being provided to students who are deaf and hard of hearing.

Audiogram Interpretation Exercises

PATIENT 1

J.J., a 9-year-old male, was seen for an audiologic evaluation after an ATV accident several weeks ago that resulted in a head injury. He sustained a concussion after his ATV rolled over on a dirt road. Fortunately, he was wearing a helmet. He stated that after the accident his right ear was bleeding. Since that time J.J. has had problems hearing in his right ear. He also reported intermittent pain on the right side of his head and also in his ear. Prior to the time of the ATV accident J.J. was in excellent health. The remainder of his medical history is unremarkable.

1. What information in the patient's case history is of concern to you?

2. Describe the hearing sensitivity in each ear.

3. What might be the reason for the hearing loss in the right ear?

4. Describe the patient's speech recognition results in each ear.

5. Describe the immittance results in each ear.

6. What is the possible etiology of the hearing loss in the right ear?

7. What recommendations do you have for this patient?

NAME: Patient 1   AGE/DATE OF BIRTH: 9 y/o

REFERRED BY: _____   MEDICAL RECORD #: _____

TEST INTERVAL: _____   DATE OF TEST: _____

PURE TONE AUDIOMETRY (RE: ANSI 1996)

KEY:

LEFT	STIMULUS	RIGHT
X	AIR	O
☐	AIR - MASK	△
>	BONE	<
]	BONE - MASK	[
↘	NO RESPONSE	↙
L	AIDED SOUND FIELD	R
	SOUND FIELD = S	

TEST TYPE
STANDARD CAE
PLAY
COR/VRA
BOA

TRANSDUCER
INSERT
CIRCUMAURAL
SOUND FIELD

RELIABILITY
EXCELLENT
GOOD
FAIR
POOR

BOOTH
#1
#2 (PEDS)
#3
#4 COCH IMPLANT

TYMPANOMETRY (226 Hz)

EAR	LEFT	RIGHT
STATIC ADMITTANCE (mm H$_2$O)		
TYMP PEAK PRESSURE (DaPa)		
TYMP WIDTH (DaPa)		
EAR CANAL VOLUME cm^3	.47	1.4

LEFT — Admittance — Pressure

RIGHT — Admittance — Pressure

CONTRA	.5k Hz	1k Hz	2k Hz	4k Hz	IPSI	.5k Hz	1k Hz	2k Hz	4k Hz
Right (AD) (phone ear)	NR	NR	NR	NR	AD (probe ear)	NR	NR	NR	
Left (AS) (phone ear)	90	95	90	NR	AS (probe ear)	95	90	95	

MIDDLE EAR ANALYZER _____

SPEECH AUDIOMETRY

	PTA	SRT/SAT	Speech Recognition	Speech Recognition	MCL	UCL
RIGHT (AD)	40	40	92 %	80	%	
Masking				50		
LEFT (AS)	12	10	100 %	50	%	
Masking				50		

MLV ☐	CD/tape ☒	W-22 ☒	WIPI ☐	PBK ☐	SPECIAL:	SPECIAL:
SOUND FIELD			%		%	
RIGHT AIDED			%		%	
LEFT AIDED			%		%	
BINAURAL			%		%	

OTOACOUSTIC EMISSIONS (OAEs)

EMISSION TYPE USED	TEST TYPE PERFORMED
☒ Transient	☒ OAE Complete
☐ Distortion Product	☐ OAE Screening

OAE results:

Right Ear   Present

Left Ear   Present

OAE UNIT _____

HEARING AID INFORMATION

RIGHT AID: _____

LEFT AID: _____

OTOSCOPY: _____

HISTORY/IMPRESSIONS/RECOMMENDATIONS: _____

_____

_____

_____

_____

_____

AUDIOLOGIST: _____   ASSISTANT: _____   AUDIOMETER: _____

FIGURE 2.2   Patient 1

PATIENT 2

C., a 9-year-old male, was seen for an audiological evaluation. C. is in third grade and overall is doing very well as reported by his mother. He was diagnosed with ADHD at the age of 4 years. Since that time, he has been taking stimulant medication for the ADHD. His mother reports that overall he is doing well on the medication with minimal side effects. His teacher is concerned that he may have a hearing problem, as it appears at times that he is not "listening" to her and has difficulty following verbal directions. There is a family history on the father's side of ADHD, learning disabilities, and auditory processing problems. The remainder of C.'s medical history is unremarkable.

1. What is the relationship between ADHD and APD?

2. What are some possible signs of APD involvement?

3. Describe the pure tone test results in each ear.

4. Describe the speech audiometric results in each ear.

5. What type of immittance results would you expect in each ear? Provide a rationale for your response.

6. What additional recommendations would you make?

NAME: Patient 2

AGE/DATE OF BIRTH: 9 y/o

REFERRED BY: _____

MEDICAL RECORD #: _____

TEST INTERVAL: _____

DATE OF TEST: _____

PURE TONE AUDIOMETRY (RE: ANSI 1996)

KEY:

LEFT	STIMULUS	RIGHT
X	AIR	O
☐	AIR - MASK	Δ
>	BONE	<
]	BONE - MASK	[
↘	NO RESPONSE	✓
L	AIDED SOUND FIELD	R
	SOUND FIELD = S	

TEST TYPE
- STANDARD CAE
- PLAY
- COR/VRA
- BOA

TRANSDUCER
- INSERT
- CIRCUMAURAL
- SOUND FIELD

RELIABILITY
- EXCELLENT
- GOOD
- FAIR
- POOR

BOOTH
- #1
- #2 (PEDS)
- #3
- #4 COCH IMPLANT

TYMPANOMETRY (226 Hz)

EAR	LEFT	RIGHT
STATIC ADMITTANCE (mm H2O)		
TYMP PEAK PRESSURE (DaPa)		
TYMP WIDTH (DaPa)		
EAR CANAL VOLUME cm3		

LEFT | RIGHT

Admittance

Pressure | Pressure

CONTRA	.5k Hz	1k Hz	2k Hz	4k Hz	IPSI	.5k Hz	1k Hz	2k Hz	4k Hz
Right (AD) (phone ear)					AD (probe ear)				
Left (AS) (phone ear)					AS (probe ear)				

MIDDLE EAR ANALYZER _____

SPEECH AUDIOMETRY

	PTA	SRT/SAT	Speech Recognition		Speech Recognition		MCL	UCL
RIGHT (AD)	0	5	100 %	45	%			
Masking								
LEFT (AS)	0	0	100 %	40	%			
Masking								

	MLV	CD/tape	W-22	WIPI	PBK	SPECIAL:	SPECIAL:
	☒	☐	☐	☐	☒		
SOUND FIELD			%		%		
RIGHT AIDED			%		%		
LEFT AIDED			%		%		
BINAURAL			%		%		

OTOACOUSTIC EMISSIONS (OAEs)

EMISSION TYPE USED	TEST TYPE PERFORMED
Transient	OAE Complete
Distortion Product	OAE Screening

OAE results:

Right Ear

Left Ear

OAE UNIT _____

HEARING AID INFORMATION

RIGHT AID: _____

LEFT AID: _____

OTOSCOPY: _____

HISTORY/IMPRESSIONS/RECOMMENDATIONS: _____

_____

_____

_____

_____

_____

AUDIOLOGIST: _____ ASSISTANT: _____ AUDIOMETER: _____

FIGURE 2.3 Patient 2

PATIENT 3

S., a 14-year-old female, was seen for a follow-up audiological evaluation to monitor her hearing sensitivity. She had a history of a cholesteatoma in her right ear, which was surgically removed five years ago. At the time of surgery it was found that her stapes had degenerated as a result of untreated chronic otitis media. The otologist performed a stapedectomy and replaced the stapes with a prosthetic device. S. has reported improvement in her hearing as a result of the surgery. S. reports no academic, social, or emotional problems as a result of the hearing loss in her right ear. Previous audiological test results from a year ago suggested a mild-to-moderate conductive hearing loss in the right ear with air-bone gaps of 15 dB HL across frequencies. Test results suggest normal hearing sensitivity in the left ear.

1. Describe the patient's hearing sensitivity in each ear.

2. Is masking necessary for air and/or bone conduction? in the right ear?

3. What are the results of the OAEs?

4. What are two audiologic recommendations you would make for this patient?

NAME: ___Patient 3___   AGE/DATE OF BIRTH: __14 y/o__

REFERRED BY: _____   MEDICAL RECORD #: _____

TEST INTERVAL: _____   DATE OF TEST: _____

PURE TONE AUDIOMETRY (RE: ANSI 1996)

KEY:

LEFT	STIMULUS	RIGHT
X	AIR	O
□	AIR - MASK	Δ
>	BONE	<
]	BONE - MASK	[
↘	NO RESPONSE	✓
L	AIDED SOUND FIELD	R

SOUND FIELD = S

TEST TYPE
STANDARD CAE
PLAY
COR/VRA
BOA

TRANSDUCER
INSERT
CIRCUMAURAL
SOUND FIELD

RELIABILITY
EXCELLENT
GOOD
FAIR
POOR

BOOTH
#1
#2 (PEDS)
#3
#4 COCH IMPLANT

TYMPANOMETRY (226 Hz)

EAR	LEFT	RIGHT
STATIC ADMITTANCE (mm H₂O)		
TYMP PEAK PRESSURE (DaPa)		
TYMP WIDTH (DaPa)		
EAR CANAL VOLUME cm³	.72	CNT

LEFT   RIGHT   DNT

Admittance   Pressure   Pressure

CONTRA	5k Hz	1k Hz	2k Hz	4k Hz	IPSI	5k Hz	1k Hz	2k Hz	4k Hz
Right (AD) (phone ear)					AD (probe ear)				
Left (AS) (phone ear)	DNT				AS (probe ear)	DNT			

MIDDLE EAR ANALYZER _____

SPEECH AUDIOMETRY

	PTA	SRT/SAT	Speech Recognition		Speech Recognition		MCL	UCL
RIGHT (AD)	40	35	100 %	75	%			
Masking				50				
LEFT (AS)	0	5	100 %	45	%			
Masking								

MLV □	CD/tape ☒	W-22 ☒	WIPI □	PBK □	SPECIAL:		SPECIAL:
SOUND FIELD		%		%			
RIGHT AIDED		%		%			
LEFT AIDED		%		%			
BINAURAL		%		%			

OTOACOUSTIC EMISSIONS (OAEs)

EMISSION TYPE USED	TEST TYPE PERFORMED
☒ Transient	☒ OAE Complete
Distortion Product	OAE Screening

OAE results:

Right Ear   Absent

Left Ear   Present

OAE UNIT _____

HEARING AID INFORMATION

RIGHT AID: _____

LEFT AID: _____

OTOSCOPY: _____

HISTORY/IMPRESSIONS/RECOMMENDATIONS: _Did not test tympanogram in right ear due to surgery._

_____

_____

_____

_____

_____

AUDIOLOGIST: _____   ASSISTANT: _____   AUDIOMETER: _____

FIGURE 2.4   Patient 3

Audiogram Interpretation Exercises

PATIENT 4

K., a 5-year-old female, was seen for an audiological reevaluation following hospitalization for meningitis. She was previously seen at this clinic two weeks ago. At that time, the results of the audiological evaluation revealed a severe-to-profound sensorineural hearing loss bilaterally with minimal speech understanding ability. Immittance results suggested normal middle-ear functioning bilaterally.

Up to the time of contracting meningitis, K. appeared to have normal hearing; she passed several preschool hearing screenings. She has no history of otitis media or speech and language problems. K. appeared lethargic during the evaluation and did not respond when spoken to by the audiologist. Prior to meningitis, K. had no medical problems. At present, she is being seen by Occupational Therapy to assess her fine motor abilities, as they appear to have diminished since the meningitis. K. was enrolled in kindergarten but was not attending school due to her poor health status.

1. What is the typical impact of meningitis on the auditory mechanism?

2. Describe the child's hearing loss.

3. Why was word recognition testing not performed?

4. Describe the tympanogram in each ear.

5. Why are the contralateral and ipslateral reflexes not measurable in each ear?

6. What are some audiologic recommendations that you would make for this child and her family?

NAME: _Patient 4_   AGE/DATE OF BIRTH: _5 y/o_

REFERRED BY: _____   MEDICAL RECORD #: _____

TEST INTERVAL: _____   DATE OF TEST: _____

PURE TONE AUDIOMETRY (RE: ANSI 1996)

KEY:

	Left	Right
Air	X	O
Air Mask	□	△
Bone	>	<
Bone - Mask	]	[
No Response	↘	↙
Aided Sound Field	A	A
Sound Field	S	S

TEST TYPE
- Standard OAE
- Play
- COR/VRA
- BOA

TRANSDUCER
- Insert
- Circumaural
- Sound Field

RELIABILITY
- Excellent
- Good
- Fair
- Poor

BOOTH
- #1
- #2
- Non-Occluded

TYMPANOMETRY (226 Hz)

EAR	LEFT	RIGHT
STATIC ADMITTANCE (mm H₂O)		
TYMP PEAK PRESSURE (DaPa)		
TYMP WIDTH (DaPa)		
EAR CANAL VOLUME cm³	.60	.54

LEFT   RIGHT   Admittance
Pressure   Pressure

CONTRA	5k Hz	1k Hz	2k Hz	4k Hz	IPSI	5k Hz	1k Hz	2k Hz	4k Hz
Right (AD) (phone ear)	NR	NR	NR	NR	AD (probe ear)	NR	NR	NR
Left (AS) (phone ear)	NR	NR	NR	NR	AS (probe ear)	NR	NR	NR

MIDDLE EAR ANALYZER _____

SPEECH AUDIOMETRY

	PTA	SRT/SAT	Speech Recognition	Speech Recognition	MCL	UCL
Right (AD)		90	CNT %	%		
Masking						
Left (AS)		90	CNT %	%		
Masking						

MLV	CID	W-22	WIPI	PBK	SPECIAL	SPECIAL
	□	□	□			
SOUND FIELD			%	%		
RIGHT AIDED			%	%		
LEFT AIDED			%	%		
BINAURAL			%	%		

OTOACOUSTIC EMISSIONS (OAEs)

EMISSION TYPE USED	TEST TYPE PERFORMED
Transient	OAE Complete
Distortion Product	OAE Screening
OAE results:	
Right Ear	
Left Ear	

OAE UNIT _____

HEARING AID INFORMATION

RIGHT AID: _____

LEFT AID: _____

OTOSCOPY: _____

HISTORY/IMPRESSIONS/RECOMMENDATIONS: _SRT obtained with selected spondee word list due to severity of loss bilaterally_

_____

_____

_____

_____

AUDIOLOGIST: _____   ASSISTANT: _____   AUDIOMETER: _____

FIGURE 2.5 Patient 4

PATIENT 5

D., a 12-year-old female, was seen for an audiological evaluation. At this time, D. is experiencing a great deal of academic difficulties. She has stated that she has problems understanding speech in the classroom, in noise, and on the telephone. D. is experiencing difficulty especially in the areas of reading and language comprehension. D. failed the sixth grade last year. D. had a hearing screening two years ago, which she passed in both ears. She had a bout of the mumps last year that she believes affected her hearing in the left ear.

1. What information in the case history may indicate the presence of a hearing loss?

2. What are the results of the unmasked air conduction thresholds in each ear?

3. What are the results of the masked air and bone conduction thresholds in the left ear?

4. Why were there initial responses to air and bone conduction testing in the unmasked condition in the left ear?

5. What speech audiometric results would you expect for the left ear?

6. What would the OAE results be for this patient?

7. What type of academic problems and communication problems would you expect in each ear?

relationship btwn air + bone

one ear = fine
one ear = not
asymmetrical
hearing

NAME: Patient 5

REFERRED BY: _Anne Sullivan_

TEST INTERVAL: _____

AGE/DATE OF BIRTH: _12 y/o_

MEDICAL RECORD #: _____

DATE OF TEST: _1890_

PURE TONE AUDIOMETRY (RE: ANSI 1996)

bone
normal

more than 40 db diff = air

if 40 db needs to be masked + use broadband noise in one ear

test for masking when air conduction between RTL

masked bone conduction

high as equip can go

KEY:

LEFT	STRADDLE	RIGHT	
X		O	AIR
☐		Δ	AIR - MASK
>		<	BONE
[		]	BONE - MASK
↘		↙	NO RESPONSE
		✓	AIDED
L	SOUND FIELD	R	

SOUND FIELD = S

TEST TYPE
STANDARD CAE
PLAY
COR/VRA
BOA

TRANSDUCER
INSERT
CIRCUMAURAL
SOUND FIELD

RELIABILITY
EXCELLENT
GOOD
FAIR
POOR

BOOTH
#1
#2 (PEDS)
#3
#4 COCH IMPLANT

TYMPANOMETRY (226 Hz)

EAR	LEFT	RIGHT
STATIC ADMITTANCE (mm H₂O)		
TYMP PEAK PRESSURE (DaPa)		
TYMP WIDTH (DaPa)		
EAR CANAL VOLUME cm³	.47	.44

LEFT | RIGHT
Admittance
Pressure | Pressure

CONTRA	.5k Hz	1k Hz	2k Hz	4k Hz	IPSI	.5k Hz	1k Hz	2k Hz	4k Hz
Right (AD) (phone ear)					AD (probe ear)				
Left (AS) (phone ear)					AS (probe ear)				

MIDDLE EAR ANALYZER _____

OTOACOUSTIC EMISSIONS (OAEs)

EMISSION TYPE USED	TEST TYPE PERFORMED
Transient	OAE Complete
Distortion Product	OAE Screening
OAE results:	
Right Ear Present	
Left Ear Absent	

OAE UNIT _____

SPEECH AUDIOMETRY

	PTA	SRT/SAT	Speech Recognition	Speech Recognition	MCL	UCL
RIGHT (AD)	6	10	100 %	%		
Masking						
LEFT (AS)	CNT	CNT	CNT %	%		
Masking						

MLV ☐	CD/tape ☒	W-22 ☒	WIPI ☐	PBK ☐	SPECIAL:	SPECIAL:
SOUND FIELD			%		%	
RIGHT AIDED			%		%	
LEFT AIDED			%		%	
BINAURAL			%		%	

HEARING AID INFORMATION

RIGHT AID: _____

LEFT AID: _____

OTOSCOPY: _____

degree car or degree masking. do book examples

HISTORY/IMPRESSIONS/RECOMMENDATIONS: _New left ear, become bff w/ helen keller_

_____

_____

_____

_____

AUDIOLOGIST: _Nielle Berens_ ASSISTANT: _Elliott Glass_ AUDIOMETER: _Evan Kolisnick_

FIGURE 2.6 Patient 5

Audiogram Interpretation Exercises

PATIENT 6

B., a 13-year-old male, was seen for an audiological evaluation. He was referred by his school psychologist. B. has reported that he cannot hear in both ears. At present, B. is having academic problems and is failing some classes. His home situation is very unstable due to his parents' recent separation. He has two younger siblings at home whom he takes care of while his mother is working in the late afternoon. Prior to his parents' separation, B. was an A student and active in sports. At present, mom reports that he appears to be withdrawn, depressed, and isolated and is not interested in activities that he pursued in the past. During the evaluation, B. strained to hear, making facial grimaces, closely watching the audiologist's lips, cupping his ear, and pressing on the earphones when auditory stimuli were presented.

1. What are some inconsistencies in the audiologic test results?

2. What are some concerns that you may have related to the patient's behavior during the case history intake and the test session?

3. What additional tests would you recommend for this patient?

4. What do you think that the patient's true thresholds might be?

5. What are two recommendations that you would make for this child and his family?

NAME: Patient 6   AGE/DATE OF BIRTH: 13 y/o

REFERRED BY: _____   MEDICAL RECORD #: _____

TEST INTERVAL: _____   DATE OF TEST: _____

PURE TONE AUDIOMETRY (RE: ANSI 1996)

KEY:

	STIMULUS	
LEFT		RIGHT
X	AIR	O
☐	AIR - MASK	Δ
>	BONE	<
]	BONE - MASK	[
↘	NO RESPONSE	✓
L	AIDED SOUND FIELD	R
	SOUND FIELD = S	

TEST TYPE
STANDARD CAE
PLAY
COR/VRA
BOA

TRANSDUCER
INSERT
CIRCUMAURAL
SOUND FIELD

RELIABILITY
EXCELLENT
GOOD
FAIR
POOR

BOOTH
#1
#2 (PEDS)
#3
#4 COCH IMPLANT

TYMPANOMETRY (226 Hz)

EAR	LEFT	RIGHT
STATIC ADMITTANCE (mm H₂O)		
TYMP PEAK PRESSURE (DaPa)		
TYMP WIDTH (DaPa)		
EAR CANAL VOLUME cm³	.83	.87

LEFT   RIGHT
Pressure   Pressure

CONTRA	5k Hz	1k Hz	2k Hz	4k Hz	IPSI	5k Hz	1k Hz	2k Hz	4k Hz
Right (AD) (phone ear)	90	95	85	90	AD (probe ear)	85	90	95	
Left (AS) (phone ear)	90	95	90	✕	AS (probe ear)	85	85	90	

MIDDLE EAR ANALYZER _____

SPEECH AUDIOMETRY

	PTA	SRT/SAT	Speech Recognition	Speech Recognition	MCL	UCL
RIGHT (AD)	50	15	100 %	55 dBHL	%	
Masking						
LEFT (AS)	50	15	100 %	55 dBHL	%	
Masking						

MLV ☒	CD/tape ☐	W-22 ☒	WIPI ☐	PBK ☐	SPECIAL:	SPECIAL:
SOUND FIELD			%	%		
RIGHT AIDED			%	%		
LEFT AIDED			%	%		
BINAURAL			%	%		

OTOACOUSTIC EMISSIONS (OAEs)

EMISSION TYPE USED	TEST TYPE PERFORMED
☒ Transient	OAE Complete
Distortion Product	☒ OAE Screening

OAE results:

Right Ear	Present
Left Ear	Present

OAE UNIT _____

HEARING AID INFORMATION

RIGHT AID: _____

LEFT AID: _____

OTOSCOPY: _____

HISTORY/IMPRESSIONS/RECOMMENDATIONS: Patient exhibited exaggeraed behavrios during the audiological evaluation inclyding pushing earphones close to head and facial grimmaces. _____

_____

_____

_____

AUDIOLOGIST: _____   ASSISTANT: _____   AUDIOMETER: _____

FIGURE 2.7   Patient 6

Audiogram Interpretation Exercises

A.B., a 5-month-old infant who failed the hearing screening prior to discharge from the hospital, was seen for a follow-up audiologic evaluation. Prenatal, perinatal, and postnatal histories were unremarkable. There is no family history of hearing loss. Parents reported that A.B. does not babble and appears not to respond to sounds in the environment. Parents expressed concerns about their daughter's hearing. As this is their first child, they are not sure what to expect with regard to speech-language-hearing milestones. DPOAEs were absent bilaterally. ABR responses were not measurable in both ears. Tympanograms suggested normal middle-ear pressure with normal tympanic membrane mobility bilaterally. Contralateral and ipsilateral acoustic reflexes were not measurable bilaterally. These test results were obtained under sedation.

1. Based on the audiologic data collected to date, what degree of hearing loss do you think the infant may have?

2. What additional tests might you recommend?

3. What would be your next steps with regard to audiologic rehabilitation for this infant?

4. What might be an additional recommendation if the child does not show significant improvement with the hearing aids and FM system?

NAME: Patient 7   AGE/DATE OF BIRTH: 5 months

REFERRED BY: _____   MEDICAL RECORD #: _____

TEST INTERVAL: _____   DATE OF TEST: _____

PURE TONE AUDIOMETRY (RE: ANSI 1996)

HEARING LEVEL IN DECIBELS (dB) — frequencies: 250, 500, 1000, 2000, 4000, 8000

SPEECH FREQUENCIES — 250, 4000, 8000

KEY:

LEFT	STIMULUS	RIGHT
X	AIR	O
☐	AIR - MASK	Δ
>	BONE	<
]	BONE - MASK	[
↘	NO RESPONSE	✓
L	AIDED SOUND FIELD	R
	SOUND FIELD = S	

TEST TYPE
STANDARD CAE
PLAY
COR/VRA
BOA

TRANSDUCER
INSERT
CIRCUMAURAL
SOUND FIELD

RELIABILITY
EXCELLENT
GOOD
FAIR
POOR

BOOTH
#1
#2 (PEDS)
#3
#4 COCH IMPLANT

TYMPANOMETRY (226 Hz)

EAR	LEFT	RIGHT
STATIC ADMITTANCE (mm H₂O)		
TYMP PEAK PRESSURE (DaPa)		
TYMP WIDTH (DaPa)		
EAR CANAL VOLUME cm³	.40	.54

LEFT — Admittance / Pressure

RIGHT — Admittance / Pressure

CONTRA	5k Hz	1k Hz	2k Hz	4k Hz	IPSI	.5k Hz	1k Hz	2k Hz	4k Hz
Right (AD) (phone ear)					AD (probe ear)				
Left (AS) (phone ear)	CNT				AS (probe ear)	CNT			

MIDDLE EAR ANALYZER _____

SPEECH AUDIOMETRY

	PTA	SRT/SAT	Speech Recognition	Speech Recognition	MCL	UCL
RIGHT (AD)			%	%		
Masking						
LEFT (AS)			%	%		
Masking						

MLV ☒	CD/tape ☐	W-22 ☐	WIPI ☐	PBK ☐	SPECIAL:	SPECIAL:
SOUND FIELD		SAT 35dBHL	%	%		
RIGHT AIDED			%	%		
LEFT AIDED			%	%		
BINAURAL			%	%		

OTOACOUSTIC EMISSIONS (OAEs)

EMISSION TYPE USED	TEST TYPE PERFORMED
Transient	OAE Complete
Distortion Product	OAE Screening

OAE results:

Right Ear   Absent

Left Ear   Absent

OAE UNIT _____

HEARING AID INFORMATION

RIGHT AID: _____

LEFT AID: _____

OTOSCOPY: _____

HISTORY/IMPRESSIONS/RECOMMENDATIONS: ABR waves were not present in both ears.

Could not test acoustic reflexes due to excessive movement.

_____

_____

_____

_____

AUDIOLOGIST: _____   ASSISTANT: _____   AUDIOMETER: _____

FIGURE 2.8 Patient 7

R., a 2-year-old female, was referred for an audiologic evaluation by her developmental pediatrician. R. passed a neonatal hearing screening conducted right after birth. At the time of this evaluation she appeared to have significant developmental delays in cognition, gross and fine motor skills, and speech-language development. There were no significant prenatal, perinatal, or postnatal histories. Over the last several months, her developmental pediatrician has shown concern regarding R.'s hearing status. In addition, R. has recently developed vision problems. Despite physical therapy, occupational therapy, and speech-language therapy, R. has demonstrated minimal improvement in developmental milestones. A referral has been made for genetic testing as well as blood tests. It is suspected that the infant may have a cytomegalovirus (CMV) infection because the mother tested positive for CMV during pregnancy. There is no history of hearing loss in the family.

1. What is the relationship between CMV and hearing loss?

2. Based on the three audiograms from the last two years, describe the changes in hearing status.

3. Why do you think there has been a significant change in the child's hearing loss over a one-year period?

4. What changes would you make in the audiologic rehabilitation plan for R.?

5. What audiologic recommendations would you make?

NAME: Patient 8-A

AGE/DATE OF BIRTH: 2 y/o

REFERRED BY: _____

MEDICAL RECORD #: _____

TEST INTERVAL: _____

DATE OF TEST: _____

PURE TONE AUDIOMETRY (RE: ANSI 1996)

KEY:

LEFT	STIMULUS	RIGHT
X	AIR	O
□	AIR - MASK	△
>	BONE	<
]	BONE - MASK	[
↘	NO RESPONSE	✓
L	AIDED SOUND FIELD	R
	SOUND FIELD = S	

TEST TYPE
- STANDARD OAE
- PLAY
- COR/VRA
- BOA

TRANSDUCER
- INSERT
- CIRCUMAURAL
- SOUND FIELD

RELIABILITY
- EXCELLENT
- GOOD
- FAIR
- POOR

BOOTH
- #1
- #2 (PEDS)
- #3
- #4 COCH IMPLANT

TYMPANOMETRY (226 Hz)

EAR	LEFT	RIGHT
STATIC ADMITTANCE (mm H$_2$O)		
TYMP PEAK PRESSURE (DaPa)		
TYMP WIDTH (DaPa)		
EAR CANAL VOLUME cm^3	.42	.88

LEFT — Admittance / Pressure

RIGHT — Admittance / Pressure

CONTRA	5k Hz	1k Hz	2k Hz	4k Hz	IPSI	5k Hz	1k Hz	2k Hz	4k Hz
Right (AD) (phone ear)					AD (probe ear)				
Left (AS) (phone ear)					AS (probe ear)				

MIDDLE EAR ANALYZER _____

SPEECH AUDIOMETRY

	PTA	SRT/SAT	Speech Recognition	Speech Recognition	MCL	UCL
RIGHT (AD)		25	%	%		
Masking						
LEFT (AS)		20	%	%		
Masking						

MLV	CD/tape ☐	W-22 ☐	WIPI ☐	PBK ☐	SPECIAL:	SPECIAL: Body Parts
SOUND FIELD			%		%	
RIGHT AIDED			%		%	
LEFT AIDED			%		%	
BINAURAL			%		%	

OTOACOUSTIC EMISSIONS (OAEs)

EMISSION TYPE USED	TEST TYPE PERFORMED
Transient	OAE Complete
Distortion Product	OAE Screening
OAE results:	
Right Ear Present	
Left Ear Present	

OAE UNIT _____

HEARING AID INFORMATION

RIGHT AID: _____

LEFT AID: _____

OTOSCOPY: _____

HISTORY/IMPRESSIONS/RECOMMENDATIONS: ABR thresholds for Wave V were present at 20dBHL in the left ear and 25dBHL in the right ear. _____

_____

_____

_____

_____

AUDIOLOGIST: _____   ASSISTANT: _____   AUDIOMETER: _____

FIGURE 2.9A   Patient 8, Audiogram 1

Audiogram Interpretation Exercises

PURE TONE AUDIOMETRY (RE: ANSI 1996)

KEY

LEFT	STIMULUS	RIGHT
X	AIR	O
☐	AIR - MASK	Δ
>	BONE	<
]	BONE - MASK	[
↘	NO RESPONSE	✓
L	AIDED SOUND FIELD	R
	SOUND FIELD = S	

TEST TYPE
| STANDARD / CAE |
| PLAY |
| COR/VRA |
| BOA |

TRANSDUCER
| INSERT |
| CIRCUMAURAL |
| SOUND FIELD |

RELIABILITY
| EXCELLENT |
| GOOD |
| FAIR |
| POOR |

BOOTH
| #1 |
| #2 (PEDS) |
| #3 |
| #4 COCH IMPLANT |

TYMPANOMETRY (226 Hz)

EAR	LEFT	RIGHT
STATIC ADMITTANCE (mm H₂O)		
TYMP PEAK PRESSURE (DaPa)		
TYMP WIDTH (DaPa)		
EAR CANAL VOLUME cm³	.92	.88

LEFT   Admittance   RIGHT

Pressure   Pressure

CONTRA	.5k Hz	1k Hz	2k Hz	4k Hz	IPSI	.5k Hz	1k Hz	2k Hz	4k Hz
Right (AD) (phone ear)					AD (probe ear)				
Left (AS) (phone ear)					AS (probe ear)				

MIDDLE EAR ANALYZER _____

SPEECH AUDIOMETRY

	PTA	SRT/SAT	Speech Recognition	Speech Recognition	MCL	UCL
RIGHT (AD)		45	%	%		
Masking						
LEFT (AS)		70	%	%		
Masking						

MLV ☒	CD/tape ☐	W-22 ☐	WIPI ☐	PBK ☐	SPECIAL:	SPECIAL: Body Parts
SOUND FIELD			%		%	
RIGHT AIDED			%		%	
LEFT AIDED			%		%	
BINAURAL			%		%	

OTOACOUSTIC EMISSIONS (OAEs)

EMISSION TYPE USED	TEST TYPE PERFORMED
Transient	OAE Complete
Distortion Product	OAE Screening

OAE results:	
Right Ear	Absent
Left Ear	Absent

OAE UNIT _____

HEARING AID INFORMATION

RIGHT AID: _____

LEFT AID: _____

OTOSCOPY: _____

HISTORY/IMPRESSIONS/RECOMMENDATIONS: ABR threshold for Wave V was present at 60dBHL in the left ear and 65dBHL for the right ear.

AUDIOLOGIST: _____ ASSISTANT: _____ AUDIOMETER: _____

FIGURE 2.9B   Patient 8, Audiogram 2

NAME: Patient 8-C

AGE/DATE OF BIRTH: 2 y/o

REFERRED BY: _____

MEDICAL RECORD #: _____

TEST INTERVAL: _____

DATE OF TEST: _____

PURE TONE AUDIOMETRY (RE: ANSI 1996)

KEY:		
LEFT	**Stimulus**	**RIGHT**
X	AIR	O
□	AIR - MASK	Δ
>	BONE	<
]	BONE - MASK	[
↘	NO RESPONSE	↙
L	AIDED SOUND FIELD	R
	SOUND FIELD = S	

TEST TYPE
STANDARD	CAE
PLAY	
COR/VRA	
BOA	

TRANSDUCER
INSERT	
CIRCUMAURAL	
SOUND FIELD	

RELIABILITY
EXCELLENT	
GOOD	
FAIR	
POOR	

BOOTH
#1	
#2 (PEDS)	
#3	
#4 COCH IMPLANT	

TYMPANOMETRY (226 Hz)

EAR	LEFT	RIGHT
STATIC ADMITTANCE (mm H₂O)		
TYMP PEAK PRESSURE (DaPa)		
TYMP WIDTH (DaPa)		
EAR CANAL VOLUME cm³	.92	.88

LEFT   Admittance   RIGHT

Pressure   Pressure

CONTRA	5k Hz	1k Hz	2k Hz	4k Hz	IPSI	5k Hz	1k Hz	2k Hz	4k Hz
Right (AD) (phone ear)					AD (probe ear)				
Left (AS) (phone ear)					AS (probe ear)				

MIDDLE EAR ANALYZER _____

SPEECH AUDIOMETRY

	PTA	SRT/SAT	Speech Recognition	Speech Recognition	MCL	UCL
RIGHT (AD)			%	%		
Masking						
LEFT (AS)			%	%		
Masking						

MLV □	CD/tape □	W-22 □	WIPI □	PBK □	SPECIAL:	SPECIAL:
SOUND FIELD			%	%		
RIGHT AIDED			%	%		
LEFT AIDED			%	%		
BINAURAL			%	%		

OTOACOUSTIC EMISSIONS (OAEs)

EMISSION TYPE USED	TEST TYPE PERFORMED
Transient	OAE Complete
Distortion Product	OAE Screening
OAE results:	
Right Ear Absent	
Left Ear Absent	

OAE UNIT _____

HEARING AID INFORMATION

RIGHT AID: _____

LEFT AID: _____

OTOSCOPY: _____

HISTORY/IMPRESSIONS/RECOMMENDATIONS: ABR wave V was absent in both ears at 90dBHL.

_____

_____

_____

_____

_____

AUDIOLOGIST: _____   ASSISTANT: _____   AUDIOMETER: _____

FIGURE 2.9C   Patient 8, Audiogram 3

H., a 15-year-old Hispanic male, was referred for an audiologic evaluation after failing a school hearing screening. H. stated that he has no hearing loss. H. reported that he listens to his iPod at least five hours per day. Sometimes when he takes off the iPod, he has ringing in his ears and sounds are muffled. His mother, who accompanied him to the evaluation, is concerned about how loudly he plays his iPod. She says that she can hear the sound leaking from the ear buds. In addition, H. plays in the school band on a regular basis, with daily practice sessions for which he uses no hearing protection.

1. Describe H.'s hearing sensitivity.

2. What does the audiometric configuration suggest?

3. Based on the patients case history and audiologic data, what recommendations should be made?

PURE TONE AUDIOMETRY (RE: ANSI 1996)

KEY:

LEFT	Stimulus	RIGHT
X	AIR	O
☐	AIR - MASK	△
>	BONE	<
]	BONE - MASK	[
↘	NO RESPONSE	✓
L	AIDED SOUND FIELD	R
	SOUND FIELD = S	

TEST TYPE
- STANDARD CAE
- PLAY
- COR/VRA
- BOA

TRANSDUCER
- INSERT
- CIRCUMAURAL
- SOUND FIELD

RELIABILITY
- EXCELLENT
- GOOD
- FAIR
- POOR

BOOTH
- #1
- #2 (PEDS)
- #3
- #4 COCH IMPLANT

TYMPANOMETRY (226 Hz)

EAR	LEFT	RIGHT
STATIC ADMITTANCE (mm H$_2$O)		
TYMP PEAK PRESSURE (DaPa)		
TYMP WIDTH (DaPa)		
EAR CANAL VOLUME cm^3		

LEFT   Admittance   RIGHT

Pressure   Pressure

CONTRA	5k Hz	1k Hz	2k Hz	4k Hz	IPSI	5k Hz	1k Hz	2k Hz	4k Hz
Right (AD) (phone ear)	90	90	95	85	AD (probe ear)	85	80	95	
Left (AS) (phone ear)	90	90	90	✕	AS (probe ear)	90	95	90	

MIDDLE EAR ANALYZER _____

SPEECH AUDIOMETRY

	PTA	SRT/ SAT	Speech Recognition		Speech Recognition		MCL	UCL
RIGHT (AD)	10	10	96 %	50	%	30		
Masking								
LEFT (AS)	10	10	92 %	50	%	30		
Masking								

MLV ☐	CD/tape ✕	W-22 ☐	WIPI ☐	PBK ☐	SPECIAL: Spanish Word List	SPECIAL:
SOUND FIELD		%		%		
RIGHT AIDED		%		%		
LEFT AIDED		%		%		
BINAURAL		%		%		

OTOACOUSTIC EMISSIONS (OAEs)

EMISSION TYPE USED	TEST TYPE PERFORMED
Transient	OAE Complete
Distortion Product	OAE Screening

OAE results:

Right Ear	Present
Left Ear	Present

OAE UNIT _____

HEARING AID INFORMATION

RIGHT AID: _____

LEFT AID: _____

OTOSCOPY: _____

HISTORY/IMPRESSIONS/RECOMMENDATIONS: _____

_____

_____

_____

_____

_____

AUDIOLOGIST: _____ ASSISTANT: _____ AUDIOMETER: _____

FIGURE 2.10   Patient 9

PATIENT 10

V., a 3-year-old female, was referred by her pediatrician for an audiologic evaluation due to chronic ear infections. V. had more than six ear infections in both ears over the last two years. She has been treated somewhat unsuccessfully with antibiotics for each infection. The pediatrician is concerned about the frequency of ear infections and the reliance on antibiotic treatment. Her parents are considering pressure equalization (P.E.) tubes. Past audiograms revealed a mild-to-moderate conductive hearing loss across all frequencies with flat tympanograms (Type B) bilaterally. Her parents and preschool teacher are concerned about V.'s speech and language development because she does not speak in complete sentences.

1. What type of hearing loss is present in both ears and why?

2. What type of tympanograms was obtained in each ear?

3. What would be expected for OAEs if tested?

4. What are three recommendations that you would make for this child?

NAME: Patient 10   AGE/DATE OF BIRTH: 3 y/o

REFERRED BY: _____   MEDICAL RECORD #: _____

TEST INTERVAL: _____   DATE OF TEST: _____

PURE TONE AUDIOMETRY (RE: ANSI 1996)

KEY:

LEFT	STIMULUS	RIGHT
X	AIR	O
□	AIR - MASK	△
>	BONE	<
]	BONE - MASK	[
↘	NO RESPONSE	✓
L	AIDED SOUND FIELD	R
	SOUND FIELD = S	

TEST TYPE

STANDARD CAE	
PLAY	
COR/VRA	
BOA	

TRANSDUCER

INSERT	
CIRCUMAURAL	
SOUND FIELD	

RELIABILITY

EXCELLENT	
GOOD	
FAIR	
POOR	

BOOTH

#1	
#2 (PEDS)	
#3	
#4 COCH IMPLANT	

TYMPANOMETRY (226 Hz)

EAR	LEFT	RIGHT
STATIC ADMITTANCE (mm H$_2$O)		
TYMP PEAK PRESSURE (DaPa)		
TYMP WIDTH (DaPa)		
EAR CANAL VOLUME cm^3		

LEFT   Admittance   RIGHT

Pressure   Pressure

CONTRA	5k Hz	1k Hz	2k Hz	4k Hz	IPSI	5k Hz	1k Hz	2k Hz	4k Hz
Right (AD) (phone ear)					AD (probe ear)				
Left (AS) (phone ear)					AS (probe ear)				

MIDDLE EAR ANALYZER _____

SPEECH AUDIOMETRY

	PTA	SRT/SAT	Speech Recognition		Speech Recognition		MCL	UCL
RIGHT (AD)	DNT	DNT %		%				
Masking								
LEFT (AS)	DNT	DNT %		%				
Masking								

MLV ☒	CD/tape ☐	W-22 ☐	WIPI ☒	PBK ☐	SPECIAL:		SPECIAL:	
SOUND FIELD			%		%			
RIGHT AIDED			%		%			
LEFT AIDED			%		%			
BINAURAL			%		%			

OTOACOUSTIC EMISSIONS (OAEs)

EMISSION TYPE USED	TEST TYPE PERFORMED
Transient	OAE Complete
Distortion Product	OAE Screening

OAE results:

Right Ear

Left Ear

OAE UNIT _____

HEARING AID INFORMATION

RIGHT AID: _____

LEFT AID: _____

OTOSCOPY: _____

HISTORY/IMPRESSIONS/RECOMMENDATIONS: _____

_____

_____

_____

_____

_____

AUDIOLOGIST: _____ ASSISTANT: _____ AUDIOMETER: _____

FIGURE 2.11 Patient 10

PATIENT 11

T., a 12-year-old male, was seen for an audiologic evaluation. T. has a history of otitis media in both ears since childhood. He had P.E. tubes placed in both ears several times during early childhood. T. has not had an ear infection since age 8. One month ago, T., who is a gymnast, fell and hit his head, resulting in a mild concussion. He stated that he noticed an immediate change in his hearing sensitivity in his left ear. T. has not experienced any tinnitus or dizziness. The remainder of his medical history is unremarkable.

1. Describe the audiogram results for each ear.

2. Describe the immittance findings.

3. What is the possible etiology of the hearing loss in the left ear?

4. What is the minimum masking level for pure tone thresholds 250–2000 Hz in the left ear?

NAME: Patient 11 **AGE/DATE OF BIRTH:** 12 y/o

REFERRED BY: **MEDICAL RECORD #:**

TEST INTERVAL: **DATE OF TEST:**

PURE TONE AUDIOMETRY (RE: ANSI 1996)

KEY:

LEFT	STIMULUS	RIGHT
X	AIR	O
☐	AIR - MASK	△
>	BONE	<
]	BONE - MASK	[
↘	NO RESPONSE	✓
L	AIDED SOUND FIELD	R
	SOUND FIELD = S	

TEST TYPE
- STANDARD CAE
- PLAY
- COR/VRA
- BOA

TRANSDUCER
- INSERT
- CIRCUMAURAL
- SOUND FIELD

RELIABILITY
- EXCELLENT
- GOOD
- FAIR
- POOR

BOOTH
- #1
- #2 (PEDS)
- #3
- #4 COCH IMPLANT

TYMPANOMETRY (226 Hz)

EAR	LEFT	RIGHT
STATIC ADMITTANCE (mm H₂O)		
TYMP PEAK PRESSURE (DaPa)		
TYMP WIDTH (DaPa)		
EAR CANAL VOLUME cm³		

LEFT — Pressure   RIGHT — Pressure   Admittance

CONTRA	5k Hz	1k Hz	2k Hz	4k Hz	IPSI	5k Hz	1k Hz	2k Hz	4k Hz
Right (AD) (phone ear)			**NR**		AD (probe ear)	80	80	85	NR
Left (AS) (phone ear)					AS (probe ear)	NR	NR	NR	NR

MIDDLE EAR ANALYZER _____

SPEECH AUDIOMETRY

	PTA	SRT/SAT	Speech Recognition		Speech Recognition		MCL	UCL
RIGHT (AD)		5	100 %	45 / 40dBSL	%			
Masking								
LEFT (AS)		80	20 %	90 / 10dBSL	%			
Masking								

MLV ☐	CD/tape ✗	W-22 ✗	WIPI ☐	PBK ☐	SPECIAL:	SPECIAL:

SOUND FIELD		%		%	
RIGHT AIDED		%		%	
LEFT AIDED		%		%	
BINAURAL		%		%	

OTOACOUSTIC EMISSIONS (OAEs)

EMISSION TYPE USED	TEST TYPE PERFORMED
Transient	OAE Complete
✗ Distortion Product	OAE Screening
OAE results:	
Right Ear Present	
Left Ear Absent	

OAE UNIT _____

HEARING AID INFORMATION

RIGHT AID: _____

LEFT AID: _____

OTOSCOPY: _____

HISTORY/IMPRESSIONS/RECOMMENDATIONS: _____

_____

_____

_____

_____

AUDIOLOGIST: _____ **ASSISTANT:** _____ **AUDIOMETER:** _____

FIGURE 2.12 Patient 11

Audiogram Interpretation Exercises

Clinical Enrichment Projects

1. What are some of the potential long-term effects of otitis media? Discuss the implications for clinical audiologic practice in the management of children with chronic otitis media.

2. What are the differences between attention deficit hyperactivity disorder (ADHD) and auditory processing disorder (APD)? Can the two exist together? What might be some recommendations that can be made for the pediatric population with ADHD and APD? Who are the members of the interdisciplinary team that should develop the best intervention plan for these children?

3. What are some issues that need to be considered in working with parents from culturally and linguistically diverse backgrounds in the diagnosis and rehabilitation of their child's hearing loss? What are some areas of concern that need to be kept in mind in order for audiology services to be sensitive to the communication needs of children and adults from diverse backgrounds?

4. Investigate your state's universal newborn screening program to answer the following questions:
   - When did the universal newborn screening program begin?
   - How many neonates have been screened?
   - How many have been referred for follow-up testing?
   - What is the pass/fail rate?
   - What is the cost-effectiveness of the program related to false-positive and false-negative referral rates?
   - What personnel are used in universal hearing screening and supervision?

5. What is the role of the audiologist as part of the cochlear implant team? Who are the other members of the team? What major changes have occurred in pediatric cochlear implants in terms of candidacy, assessment, and management? over the last five years?

6. What techniques can be used with young children when masking? If you cannot mask, then what tests would be used to determine the type and degree of hearing loss?

7. What is the ideal audiologic test protocol for a normally developing child of 2 or 3 years old?

8. Why is it necessary to do a combination of behavioral and electrophysiological tests on the pediatric population? How does the cross-check principle as described by Jerger and Hayes (1976) apply to testing the pediatric population?

10. Summarize the recommendations put forth by the most recent position statement by the Joint Committee on Infant Hearing (2007): *Principles and Guidelines for Early Hearing Detection and Intervention Programs.*

Answers for Audiogram Interpretation Exercises

PATIENT 1

1. *Recent ATV accident resulting in concussion and head trauma to the right side.*
2. *Normal hearing sensitivity in the left ear. Moderate flat mixed hearing loss in the right ear.*
3. *The hearing loss may be the result of concussion and head trauma. In addition, there may be disarticulation of the ossicles of the middle ear.*
4. *Excellent word recognition ability in both ears.*
5. *Tympanogram in the left ear reveals normal tympanic membrane mobility with normal middle-ear pressure (Type A). Tympanogram in the right ear reveals excessive tympanic mobility with normal middle-ear pressure (Type A$_D$). Contralateral acoustic reflexes were not measurable in both ears. Ipsilateral acoustic reflexes were measurable in the left ear and were within expected levels. Ipsilateral acoustic reflexes were not measurable in the right ear.*
6. *Head trauma with disarticulation of the ossicles.*
7. ● *Referral to ENT physician for possible medical management of hearing loss in right ear.*

PATIENT 2

1. *There is a high incidence of APD in children who have been diagnosed with ADHD.*
2. *Difficulty understanding speech in degraded conditions such as noise, difficulty following instructions, needs repetition, auditory memory problems.*
3. *Hearing sensitivity within normal limits bilaterally.*

4. *Excellent word recognition bilaterally.*
5. *Immittance results would most likely represent normal middle-ear functioning with normal expected levels.*
6. ● *Auditory processing evaluation.*

PATIENT 3

1. *Hearing sensitivity is within normal limits in the left ear. There is a mild conductive hearing loss in the right ear.*
2. *Masking is necessary for bone conduction at 250–4000 Hz; masking is not necessary for air conduction.*
3. *OAEs absent in the right ear due to presence of conductive hearing loss. OAEs are present and normal in the left ear.*
4. ● *Return to ENT physician for follow-up and audiologic annual reevaluation to monitor hearing sensitivity or sooner if otitis media returns.*

PATIENT 4

1. *Oftentimes there can be a sensorineural hearing loss ranging from mild to profound.*
2. *Severe-to-profound sensorineural hearing loss bilaterally.*
3. *Word recognition testing was not performed due to the severity of the hearing loss in both ears and the output limitations of the audiometer.*
4. *Tympanograms reveal normal middle-ear pressure with normal tympanic membrane mobility bilaterally (Type A).*

5. *They are not measurable in each ear due to the severity of the hearing loss.*
6. • *Referral for a cochlear implant evaluation for bilateral implants.*
   • *FM system.*
   • *Communication strategies training.*
   • *Counseling for family.*

PATIENT 5

1. *The bout of mumps can result in a unilateral sensorineural hearing loss. Academic problems are a concern as well due to the unilateral nature of the hearing loss and the problems that can result due to poor signal-to-noise in most classroom environments.*
2. *Normal hearing sensitivity in the right ear with a moderately severe sensorineural hearing loss in the left ear.*
3. *A profound sensorineural hearing loss in the left ear.*
4. *The initial thresholds suggesting a moderately severe hearing loss in the left ear were the result of cross hearing with the better ear responding to the pure tone stimuli.*
5. *Due to the severity of the hearing loss, speech testing could not be performed.*
6. *OAEs are present in the right ear and absent in the left ear due to the severity of the hearing loss.*
7. *Due to the unilateral hearing loss, the child may have problems with the localization of sound and problems understanding speech in noise, especially in the classroom. The child would benefit from preferential seating and an FM system used during the school day.*

PATIENT 6

1. *There is a discrepancy between the PTAs and SRTs bilaterally with the SRTs being better than PTAs. The excellent word recognition ability of the patient at 55 dB HL bilaterally would not happen given that the presentation level for the speech stimuli would be near threshold levels. The presence of OAEs bilaterally also would not be expected with the severity of the hearing loss in both ears.*
2. • *Exaggeration and straining to hear.*
   • *Focused attention of the audiologist's face for speechreading purposes.*

• *Pressing on the earphones during testing.*
   • *Parents' recent separation and unstable family life.*
3. • *ABR testing to estimate hearing threshold levels and retesting for pure times to determine the hearing thresholds.*
4. *Most likely there is no hearing loss present based on speech results and OAEs in both ears.*
5. • *Professional counseling to resolve the functional hearing loss.*

PATIENT 7

1. *The diagnostic test battery is suggestive of at least a bilateral severe sensorienural hearing loss.*
2. *Behavioral observation audiometry to corroborate the electrophysiological test results.*
3. • *Counsel the family regarding amplification.*
   • *Referral to ENT for medical clearance.*
   • *Take earmold impressions for bilateral behind-the-ear hearing aid trial.*
   • *Personal FM listening system to be used in conjunction with hearing aids.*
   • *Referral to speech-language pathologist and audiologist for early intervention program.*
   • *Encourage the family to obtain genetic counseling.*
4. *An additional recommendation might be a referral to cochlear implant team for evaluation if there is no benefit from amplification.*

PATIENT 8

1. *One in 100 infants born in the United States has active CMV. Of these, 10%–15% will develop central nervous system problems including developmental delay, intellectual deficits, and hearing loss (Northern & Downs, 2002). The hearing loss can vary in severity from a mild to profound sensorineural hearing loss that can be unilateral or bilateral. Typically, the hearing loss is progressive in nature.*
2. *Audiogram 1 suggests borderline-normal hearing in both ears. Tympanograms were consistent with normal middle-ear pressure and normal tympanic membrane mobility (Type A) bilaterally. OAEs were present bilaterally. ABR wave V thresholds suggest borderline-normal hearing sensitivity in each ear.*

Audiogram 2 was performed 6 months later. There was a significant reduction in hearing sensitivity in both ears. Pure tone conduction thresholds revealed a moderate to moderately severe hearing loss in the left ear with a severe hearing loss in the right ear. Bone conduction thresholds were not obtained at this session. Tympanograms remained the same, with normal middle-ear pressure and normal tympanic membrane mobility (Type A) bilaterally. OAEs were absent, which is probably due to the degree of hearing loss. ABR wave V threshold was present at 60 dB HL in the left ear and 65 dB HL in the right ear, suggesting a moderately severe hearing loss. Due to the significant changes in hearing sensitivity, trial use of amplification including hearing aids and FM system should be recommended. In addition, the child should be referred for early intervention services.

Audiogram 3 was completed 6 months later. The results of the tests revealed a severe-to-profound hearing loss in both ears. Tympanograms showed normal middle-ear function in both ears. OAEs were absent bilaterally. ABR wave V was absent in both ears at 90 dB HL.

3. CMV can result in a progressive sensorineural hearing loss.
4. The child will need hearing aids that are more powerful. Therapies including speech-language and early intervention should continue.
5. • Continue monitoring hearing sensitivity.
   • Possible cochlear implant evaluation.

PATIENT 9

1. Normal hearing sensitivity at 250–2000 Hz with a moderately severe to severe sensorineural hearing loss at 3000–4000 Hz, rising to a mild hearing loss at 6000–8000 Hz.
2. Noise-induced notch at 3000–4000 Hz bilaterally probably due to listening to the iPod at loud levels on a daily basis and his exposure to noise as a band member.
3. • Reduce the volume of the iPod and amount of time it is worn daily.
   • Use ear protection when exposed to loud noise such as daily band practice.
   • Audiologic evaluation annually to monitor hearing sensitivity.

PATIENT 10

1. A conductive hearing loss is present in both ears. It is a conductive loss because hearing is within normal limits for bone conduction with hearing loss present for air conduction. Air bone gaps of 20 dB HL are present across frequencies.
2. Tympanograms were flat (Type B) due to the fluid in the middle-ear system in both ears.
3. OAEs would be absent bilaterally due to the presence of conductive pathology in the middle-ear system and the mild hearing loss.
4. • Medical evaluation to determine whether P.E. tubes are a viable option.
   • Referral for speech-language diagnostic evaluation.
   • Continued follow-up with audiology; possible use of mild gain FM system in classroom or soundfield to amplify speech when a poor signal-to-noise ratio exists.

PATIENT 11

1. Hearing sensitivity within normal limits in the right ear. Severe-to-profound mixed hearing loss in the left ear.
2. Tympanogram suggested normal middle-ear pressure with normal tympanic membrane mobility in the right ear. Tympanogram suggested normal middle-ear pressure with excessive tympanic membrane mobility in the left ear (A_D). Absent contralateral and ipsilateral acoustic reflexes are consistent with a conductive component in the left ear.
3. Based on recent history of head trauma and the mixed hearing loss, the results may suggest ossicular discontinuity.
4. The minimum masking levels to eliminate cross-hearing is as follows:
   250–40 dB HL
   500–40 dB HL
   1000–60 dB HL
   2000–70 dB HL

Answers for Audiogram Interpretation Exercises

References

American Speech-Language-Hearing Association. (2005). *(Central) auditory processing disorders—The rule of the audiologist* [Position Statement]. Retrieved May 2009 from www.asha.org/policy.

Battle, D. (2002). *Communication disorders in multicultural populations* (3rd ed.). Boston: Butterworth Heinemann.

Bennett, M. J. (1984). Impedance concepts relating to the acoustic reflex. In S. Silman (Ed.), *The acoustic reflex: Basic principles and clinical applications* (pp. 35–61). New York: Academic Press.

Bess, F. H. (1985). The minimally hearing impaired child. *Ear and Hearing, 6,* 43–47.

Bess, F. H., & Tharpe, A. M. (1984). Unilateral hearing impairment in children. *Pediatrics, 74,* 206–216.

Campbell, K. (2006). *Pharmacology and ototoxicity for audiologists.* Clifton Park, NY: Delmar Cengage Learning.

Carney, A. (1996). Audition and the development of oral communication competency. In F. Bess, J. Gravel, & A. Tharpe (Eds.), *Amplification for children with auditory deficits* (pp. 29–53). Nashville, TN: Bill Wilkerson Center Press.

Chermak, G. D., Hall, J.W., III, & Musiek, F. E. (1999). Differential diagnosis and management of central auditory processing disorders and attention deficit hyperactivity disorders. *Journal of the American Academy of Audiology, 10*(6), 289–303.

Elliott, L. L. & Katz, D. R. (1980). Children's puretone detection. *Journal of the Acoustical Society of America, 67,* 342–344.

Erber, N. (1982). *Auditory training.* Washington, DC: Alexander Graham Bell Association for the Deaf.

Galvin, K. L., Mok, M., Dowell, R. C., & Briggs, R. J. (2008). Speech detection and localization results and clinical outcomes in children receiving sequential bilateral cochlear implants before four years of age. *International Journal of Audiology, 47,* 636–646.

Hall, J. (2007). *New handbook of auditory evoked responses.* Boston: Allyn & Bacon.

Hayes, D., & Northern, J. (1990). *Infants and hearing.* San Diego: Singular.

Holt, R. F., & Svirsky, M. A. (2008). An exploratory look at pediatric cochlear implantation: Is earliest always best? *Ear and Hearing 29,* (4), 492–511.

Jerger, J., & Hayes, D. (1976). The cross-check principle in pediatric audiometry. *Archives of Otolaryngology, 102,* 614–620.

Joint Committee on Infant Hearing (JCIH). (2007). Year 2007 position statement: Principles and guidelines for early hearing detection and intervention programs. *Pediatrics, 120*(4) pgs. 5–29.

Katz, J. (Ed.). (2002). *Handbook of clinical audiology* (5th ed.). Philadelphia: Lippincott Williams & Wilkins.

Kemp, D. T. (1978). Stimulated acoustic emissions from within the human auditory system. *Journal of the Acoustical Society of America, 64,* 1386–1391.

Matkin, N. D., & Wilcox, A. (1999). Considerations in the education of children with hearing loss. *Clinics of North America, 46*(1), 143–151.

McCandless, G. A., & Alfred, P. L. (1978). Tympanometry and emergence of the acoustic reflex in infants. In E. R. Harford, F. H. Bess, C. D. Bluestone, et al. (Eds.) *Impedance screening for middle ear disease in children* (pp. 56–57). New York: Grune & Staton.

National Institutes of Health (NIH). (1993). *Early identification of hearing impairment in infants and young children: NIH Consensus Development Conference statement.* Bethesda, MD: Author.

Northern, J., & Downs, M. (2002). *Hearing in children* (5th ed.). Philadelphia: Lippincott William & Wilkins.

Ross, M., & Lerman, J. (1970). A picture identification test for hearing impaired children. *Journal of Speech and Hearing Research, 13,* 43–44.

Sininger, Y. S., Hood, L. J., Starr, A., Berlin, C. I., & Picton, T. W. (1995). Hearing loss due to auditory neuropathy. *Audiology Today, 7*(2), 10–12.

Stach, B. (1999). *Clinical audiology: An introduction.* San Diego: Singular.

Recommended Readings

American Speech-Language-Hearing Association (ASHA). (1994). Joint Committee on Infant Screening 1994 position statement. *ASHA, 36,* 38–41.

Gravel, J. S., Karma, P., & Casselbrant, M. L. (2005). Recent advances in otitis media: Diagnosis and screening. *Annals of Otology and Rhinology, 194* (Laryngeal Suppl.), 103–104.

Moore, M. (2006). Hispanics may face higher risk for hearing loss from iPods and other MP3 players. *The ASHA Leader, 11*(17), 3, 17.

NIH Consensus Statement. (1993). *Early Identification of Hearing Impairments in Infants and Young Children, 11,* 1–24.

Rance, G. (2005). Auditory neurophaty/dys-synchrony and its perceptual consequences. *Trends in Amplification, 9,* 1–43.

Starr, A., Picton, T. W., Sininger, Y., Hood, L. L., & Berlin, C. I. (1996). Auditory neuropathy. *Brain, 16,* 361–371.

Yoshinaga Itano, C., Sedney, A. L., Coulter, D. K., & Mehl, A. L. (1999). Language of early and later identified children with hearing loss. *Pediatrics, 102,* 1161–1171.

Audiological Diagnosis and Management of Hearing Loss in the Older Adult Population

This section will focus on hearing loss in older adults, 60 years of age and above. Students will be required to interpret audiograms and make audiological recommendations for community-based elderly patients and nursing home residents. Information will be provided on the biological, psychological, and social factors affecting older patients and communication demands that need to be considered in providing hearing health care services to this heterogeneous population.

STUDENT LEARNING OUTCOMES

On completion of this section students will be able to:

1. Identify appropriate audiological testing protocols for community-based elderly and residents of long-term care facilities.
2. Gain an understanding of biological aging in the human body, in particular the auditory mechanism.
3. Determine the psychological aspect of hearing loss in older patients.
4. Determine the social impact of hearing loss on communication functioning in older adults.
5. Use test data to make recommendations for audiologic intervention for elderly patients.

GENERAL GUIDELINES FOR TESTING OLDER ADULTS

The following are some guidelines to keep in mind when providing audiologic services to the older population.

Guideline 1: Audiologic testing and management of hearing loss in older adults is a specialization in the profession. Audiologists who provide hearing health care services must understand the impact of the hearing loss on an older adult's lifestyle. The audiologist needs to be aware of the numerous biological, psychological, and social changes that accompany the aging process. A holistic approach needs to be followed in treating elderly adults with hearing loss.

Guideline 2: The diagnosis of hearing loss in this population is complicated. Many older adults have both a peripheral hearing loss and an auditory processing disorder. Auditory processing disorders can have significant implications on auditory management, especially related to amplification recommendations.

Guideline 3: The testing protocol for this population should include behavioral testing, a screening for auditory processing disorder, and a hearing handicap and/or communication scale. For those elderly persons who may have cognitive involvement a mental status screening should be conducted.

Guideline 4: For a variety of reasons, it may be necessary to conduct the hearing testing over several sessions, especially when dealing with aging individuals who have dementia or other cognitive impairments.

Guideline 5: Older adults residing in long-term care facilities present unique challenges to providing hearing health care services. Modification of the basic audiologic evaluation may be necessary in order to determine the hearing loss. It is critical that there be family and staff involvement to follow through with the auditory rehabilitation process.

Guideline 6: A family-centered approach is advocated when working with the aging population. This approach will provide elderly adults with the necessary support to benefit from hearing health care services. In addition, an interdisciplinary team approach may be warranted due to the numerous biological and psychosocial age-related changes. This may include a geriatrician, ophthalmologist, low-vision rehabilitation specialist, psychologist, family doctor, social worker, speech-language pathologist, physical therapist, and/or occupational therapist.

DEMOGRAPHICS OF OLDER ADULTS IN THE UNITED STATES

The fastest growing segment of the U.S. population is individuals 65 years of age and older. At present, this age group constitutes 13% of the U.S. population. By 2020, this age group will represent over 16% of the population, and by 2040, more than 20.7% of the population. The increase in longevity is due to improvements in medical technology, healthier lifestyle's, and preventive medicine. About 10 million adults who are 65 years of age and older have a hearing loss. Hearing loss has been reported to be the third most prevalent chronic health condition in the elderly (U.S. Department of Health and Human Services [U.S. DHHS], 2003).

Approximately 5% of older adults at one time in their lives will reside in a long-term care facility (Weinstein, 2000). There are several reasons why an older adult may need to reside in a long-term care facility, including (1) need for 24-hour medical care, (2) impairment in activities of daily living (ADLs), and (3) need for short-term rehabilitation. According to Weinstein (2000), about 2 million older adults in the United States reside in a long-term care facility at any given time. The highest incidence of residents are individuals 85 years and older who often have numerous acute and chronic health conditions. As the U.S. population continues to live longer, there will most likely be a greater need for more long-term care facilities over the next several decades. These frail individuals usually have a high incidence of hearing loss and cognitive impairment.

Despite whether an older adult lives in the community or in a long-term care facility, audiologic services are critical; misdiagnosed or undiagnosed hearing loss can have significant consequences on quality of life. An untreated hearing loss may lead to depression and confusion that mimic dementia. These symptoms can become worse over time if the hearing loss remains untreated. Family members and those in the health care professions need to be aware of the signs associated with hearing loss and seek services as necessary.

BIOLOGICAL CHANGES ASSOCIATED WITH AGING

This section will address some of the common biological changes and diseases associated with the aging process. Older adults tend to have numerous medical conditions. Of those over the age of 60, 40% have two or more chronic diseases; 23% of three or more; and 8% have four or more chronic conditions (Weinstein, 2000). The three most prevalent chronic health conditions are arthritis, high blood pressure, and hearing loss. Tinnitus ranks as the ninth most common chronic health condition (U.S. DHHS, 2003).

Elderly adults tend to take numerous medications for chronic health conditions, which can result in ototoxicity. It is critical that during the case history, audiologists collect data on all health conditions and medications so as to determine whether there may be an effect on the auditory and/or vestibular mechanism. It is critical that audiologists be knowledgeable about the pharmaceutical agents and the possibility of ototoxicity. Underlying diseases such as renal dysfunction can make the cochlea more susceptible to ototoxic medications. The following is a summary of some of the most significant biological changes related to the aging process.

Changes in the Nervous System

There are a variety of age-related changes that occur within the nervous system. Some of the more common include a significant reduction in brain weight that may alter the chemical composition of the brain. The number of nerve cells decreases with age (Weinstein, 2000). According to Abrams, Beers, and Berkow (1995), the loss of nerve cells may range from 10% to 60%. In some individuals, especially those with cognitive involvement such as dementia, neurofibrillary tangles may be present. Changes in the central nervous system may cause an older adult to exhibit decreases in response time and the need for more redundancy in information that is provided during hearing testing and the audiologic rehabilitation process.

Changes in the Visual System

The visual system undergoes extensive age-related changes. Many older adults will experience age-related changes in both vision and audition resulting in a dual sensory loss (Busacco, 2009). It is critical that audiologists be aware of some of the more common age-related vision changes. With normal aging, the lens of the eye becomes stiff, resulting in presbyopia (Weinstein, 2000). Presbyopia is the lack of ability of the eye to focus on objects at a normal distance. Other changes in the visual system include a yellowing of the lens resulting in a decrease in color sensitivity. Normal visual changes that accompany aging include slowed dark/light adaptation, decrease in glare recovery time, and overall decrease in color sensitivity. Some of the common eye diseases found in the elderly include cataracts, glaucoma, diabetic retinopathy, and macular degeneration (Kricos, 2007).

Visual changes and ocular diseases may prevent the older adult from using visual cues to supplement audition, such as speechreading and auditory visual speech perception. Age-related visual changes must be kept in mind when modifying the physical environment so that older adults can maximize the use of visual information to supplement audition. It is recommended that the audiologist consult with vision specialists in developing an effective auditory rehabilitation program when dual sensory loss is present (Busacco, 2009; Kricos, 2007).

Changes in the Cardiovascular System

As one ages, there are changes in the heart that can impact cardiovascular functioning. The heart increases in size, resulting in an increase in heart weight and mass. The arties of the heart stiffen with age, resulting in the heart needing to work harder to circulate blood. Aging tends to result in an increase in high blood pressure, which may affect the blood flow to the cochlea. Cardiac medications also can effect hearing and/or the vestibular mechanisms.

Changes in the Renal System

There are age-related changes in the kidneys that can impact the ability to remove wastes and toxins in the body. The kidneys tend to decrease in size and weight with age. Kidney function abnormalities may make older adults more susceptible to ototoxicity. Some drugs that are known to be ototoxic include cancer treating agents, loop diuretics, large doses of aspirin, and some mycin drugs. It is critical that older adults who are using these medications have good renal system functioning to prevent hearing loss. In addition, hearing sensitivity should be monitored over time to assess whether there are any long-term ototoxic effects.

Changes in the Immune System

Older adults tend to have declines in the body's ability to produce antibodies and in the ability to protect itself against pathogens (Weinstein, 2000). The decrease in the immune system makes older adults more susceptible to infections and autoimmune disorders such as lupus and arthritis. Some medication that can be used to treat autoimmune disease may be toxic to the auditory and/or vestibular system.

Changes in the Somatosensory System

There are age-related changes that affect the sense of touch. With aging there is a decrease in the sense of deep and light touch (Hull, 2004). This will have implications for older adults using hearing aids and/or assistive devices. Oftentimes, these individuals cannot manipulate the controls of the devices. Changes in touch sensation may necessitate selection or modifications of the amplification system to facilitate independent use of the device (e.g., automatic gain control, remote control, raised volume control) (Hull, 2004). In addition, working with an occupational therapist can be helpful in learning strategies to manipulate the amplification device (Busacco, 2009).

Changes in Cognition

With aging, there tends to be decline in cognitive functioning, including a decrease in learning and processing of new information. Older adults may need more time to process new tasks and to integrate new information. In addition, this population may have more problems in attending to several tasks at once, known as divided attention (Botwinick, 1970). Although learning capacity does not decrease with age, it may be that the elderly need to use different strategies when learning new information (Gates, Cobb, Linn, Rees, Wolf, & D'Agostino, 1996). Typically, more time is necessary for processing new information and transferring it into daily practice. This can impact the ability of the older adults to retain new information related to hearing aids (Uhlmann, Larson, Rees, Koepsell, & Duckert, 1989).

About 10% of older adults have severe cognitive involvement known as dementia (Weinstein & Amsel, 1986). Dementia is an acquired global impairment of intellectual function that interferes with the activities of daily living (ADLs). Dementia is a progressive loss of cognitive skills associated with aging. There is a relationship between dementia and hearing loss. According to Weinstein and Amsel (1986), hearing loss tends to be more prevalent in individuals with dementia and also tends to be more severe. Specific audiologic rehabilitation techniques need to be used when fitting with amplification so that quality of life is improved for the older adult and caregiver.

Changes in the Vestibular System

Older adults experience dizziness and falls on a frequent basis. Falls are the leading cause of accidental death among elderly adults age 75 years and older (DeWane, 1995). Dizziness as a result of aging of the vestibular system can significantly reduce quality of life. The vestibular system undergoes age-related changes that include degeneration of the peripheral and central vestibular system. It is beyond the scope of this book to address the numerous changes that occur in the aging vestibular system. It is critical that audiologists who perform tests of balance are aware of the age-related changes that can impact test results. When conducting a case history interview, it is mandatory that questions about dizziness, balance, and falls are addressed. When evaluating test results, it is critical that the audiologist be aware of the medications that the older patient is taking, as these can affect test outcomes. The balance protocol with this population should include, when appropriate, electronystagmography (ENG), rotational tests, and computerized posturography. Balance assessment of older adults should take an interdisciplinary approach including audiologists, neurologists, physical therapists, occupational therapists, and a geriatrician. For further information on this topic refer to (Jacobson, Newman, & Kartush, 1997).

Changes in the Auditory System

The effects of aging on the hearing mechanism are heterogeneous. Age-related changes occur in the outer, middle, and innerear, VIII nerve, auditory pathways, and the auditory cortex (Weinstein, 2000) The following is a brief overview of some age-related changes in the auditory mechanism. For extensive information on this topic refer to Weinstein (2000). Some of the age-related changes that occur in the outer ear include a thinning of the skin that covers the ear canal, thereby making it susceptible to trauma. This can have implications when conducting cerumen management and taking earmold impressions and in hearing aid usage, especially for completely-in-the-canals (CICs) that are placed deep within the ear canal. Older adults tend to have excessive cerumen that may be the result of the ear making too much cerumen or the inability of the aging ear to remove the cerumen through migration (Ballachandra, 1995). Excessive cerumen can cause a great deal of problems in providing hearing health care services to this population. Other changes that may occur in the outer ear include a loss of elasticity resulting in an elongation of the pinnae. There tends to be excessive hair growth in the ear canals in men, which can hinder the visualization of the tympanic membrane. Calcium plagues may be present on the tympanic membrane, resulting in stiffening of the tympanic membrane. The majority of age-related changes in the outer ear typically do not impact significantly on hearing sensitivity.

Age-related changes in the middle ear include a stiffening of the entire middle ear system. Although there are arthritic changes in the middle ear, the impact on hearing is minimal. In some older adults, there is atrophy and degeneration of the muscles that support the Eustachian tube, which may affect its opening and closing, resulting in Eustachian tube dysfunction. Such age-related changes typically do not impact hearing sensitivity.

The inner ear is probably the most susceptible to aging. *Presbycusis* is the term used to describe age-related changes in hearing sensitivity as evidenced in pure tone and speech audiometry. Age-related changes in the cochlea include degeneration of the organ of Corti, possible lack of blood supply to the stria vascularis, and degeneration of the outer and inner hair cells. Presbycusis will result in sensorineural hearing loss that can be amenable to audiologist intervention such as amplification.

There are numerous age-related changes in the central nervous system that can impact auditory processing ability. Some of these changes include a loss of neurons, change in the size and shape of the neurons, and a reduction in the number of dendrites (Stach, 1999). These changes vary greatly across older adults. At this time, there has not been sufficient research on this topic to document the histological changes in the brain and their impact on tests of auditory processing abilities in aging adults. Such changes in auditory processing will determine auditory rehabilitation intervention.

IMPACTS OF AGING

Impact of Aging on Audiometric Testing

A variety of studies have investigated the effects of age on pure tone behavioral thresholds (Cooper, 1994). The audiogram for women shows greater hearing loss in the low frequencies. The data from studies on men suggest that pure tone thresholds tend to be poorer in the higher frequencies, which is probably attributed to their great exposure to noise over their lifespan.

Impact of Aging on Speech Perception

Older adults typically report difficulty understanding speech in a variety of communication environments especially in the presence of background noise, reverberation, and listening at a distance. There is a great deal of heterogeneity with regard to aging and speech understanding in both quiet and noise. According to a review of the literature in Weinstein (2000), the data indicates that, when speech materials are presented at high intensity levels in quiet, older adults with hearing loss tend to perform as well as their younger counterparts. However, Gordon-Salant (1987) reported that age effects do occur for temporally altered speech materials such as time-compressed speech and that the elderly tend to perform poorly on these tests.

One condition that might be present in older adults is binaural interference. Binaural interference occurs when the binaural speech recognition ability in the aided condition is significantly poorer than the better ear aided. Testing to determine whether this condition is present includes assessment of speech understanding with hearing aids in each ear and then in the binaural condition (Jerger, Silman, Lew, & Chmiel, 1993). If binaural interference is present, then the individual may derive more benefit from using one hearing aid than two hearing aids (Walden & Walden, 2005).

Impact of Aging on Otoacoustic Emissions

The results of Harris and Probst (1997) suggest that there are no significant age effects for transient-evoked otoacoustic emissions (TEOAEs). Gorga, Neeley, Ohlrich, Hoover, Redner, and Peters (1997) reported that age does not have a significant effect on distortion-product otoacoustic emissions (DPOAEs). However, Lansbury-Martin, Martin, and Whitehead (1997) stated that age may cause a decrease in the amplitude of the DPOAEs. It could be that monitoring of OAEs for ototoxicity can be valuable in the older population especially for those taking numerous medications.

Impact of Aging on the Auditory Brainstem Response

There is controversy about the impact of aging on the auditory brainstem response. In general, the results of the ABR in older adults will be confounded by the presence of peripheral hearing loss. There are not statistically significant differences in latency and amplitude of the ABR in older adults as compared to younger counterparts (Hall, 2007). At this time there is not enough evidence to support the establishment of separate norms for older adults based on age-related changes in the peripheral auditory mechanism. This may change over time as more detailed information on older adults beyond 80 years old is obtained.

Impact of Aging on Middle Latency Response

Middle latency response is a series of waveforms that occur between 15 and 50 msec after the presentation of an acoustic stimulus. MLR waves are identified as Na, Pa, Nb, and P1. Pa is the most identifiable wave, and it occurs 25 msec after acoustic stimulation. The problem with using MLR for diagnostic testing is that the waveforms are affected by muscle artifact. Musiek and Geurhink (1981) stated that the MLR can predict hearing threshold levels in the low frequencies. There have been few studies on the effects of age on the MLR. Those studies that have been done reported that the main age effect is a reduction in the amplitude of the MLR with no significant other effects on MLR latencies (Hall, 2007).

Impact of Aging on Auditory Late Responses (ALR)

It has been well documented that aging impacts auditory late responses (ALR) especially on the amplitude and latency of the P_{300} (Hall, 2007). The P_{300} at this time is not used clinically in audiology. However, the auditory late responses may hold promise in the future to address cognitive changes in the ability to process a variety of tasks, especially speech perception. The major problem is that the older adult must be cognizant to participate in the task(s) used to assess the P_{300}.

PSYCHOSOCIAL ISSUES RELATED TO AGING

Older adults need to adjust to the many changes in their later years. Some of the psychological changes that one must deal with include the loss of family and friends, retirement, change in financial status, relocation stress, loss of identity, and diminished self-esteem (Hull, 2004). When faced with the many changes associated with getting older, there may not be a high level of motivation to pursue hearing health care services. Some elderly may be dealing with depression and issues of reduced quality of life. Bess, Lechentenstein, Logan, Burger, and Nelson (1989) noted that older adults with hearing loss tend to have a high incidence of depression and reduced perception of quality of life compared to their peers without hearing loss. These psychological changes may impact the level of motivation of this population to use hearing aids and/or assistive listening devices and pursue other forms of audiologic rehabilitation. Several hearing handicap scales have been developed specifically to address the psychosocial issues facing aging adults and the impact of hearing loss on lifestyle. One of the most commonly used hearing handicap scales is the Hearing Handicap Inventory for the Elderly (HHIE) (Weinstein & Ventry, 1983). Hearing handicap scales should be administered at different intervals throughout the audiologic rehabilitation process as outcome measurements to determine the effectiveness of intervention.

SPECIAL CONSIDERATIONS IN TESTING OLDER ADULTS

Audiological Evaluation of Nursing Home Residents

Due to the numerous physical, social, and psychological changes that nursing home residents encounter, it is probably best to provide hearing health care services at their facility. This will eliminate a great deal of difficulty with transportation to an outpatient audiologic practice. It may be necessary to modify the standard audiologic test battery when evaluating this population. For example, speech audiometry should be conducted as the initial test because some nursing home residents may not be able to follow the instructions for pure tone testing and may become easily frustrated. For those who can perform pure tone testing, it may be necessary to modify the response from hand raising to a verbal response, which is an easier task.

As a result of portable equipment, audiologic testing can be conducted at the long-term care facility, including pure tone audiometry, immittance, and otoacoustic emissions testing. Hearing aids can be dispensed to this population with a verification process that includes real ear measurements, hearing handicap scales, and hearing aid satisfaction inventories presented before and after hearing aid fitting. The major deterrent in providing audiological services to this population is the high incidence of cerumen impaction. If the audiologist is not comfortable or experienced at cerumen removal, then a medical specialist in the nursing facility should be responsible for its removal. It is critical that on admission to the facility every resident is given a hearing screening during the intake examination so that the medical staff is aware that a hearing loss exists. If untreated, hearing loss may mimic dementia or make it appear more severe (Weinstein & Amsel, 1986). As older adults live into their eighties or nineties, audiologists will be offering more hearing health care services to this frail population. Diagnostic test results should reflect the abilities of the patient, but also provide as much information about the type and degree of hearing loss so that appropriate intervention can be implemented. Hearing health care services can be delivered very effectively to this population in a cost-effective manner if all of these aforementioned factors are taken into account.

Audiologic Evaluation of Older Adults with Cognitive Impairment

Approximately 10% of older adults have some degree of cognitive impairment (Weinstein & Amsel, 1986). According to Weinstein and Amsel (1986), hearing loss is more prevalent in patients who have dementia than those without dementia. In addition, those with dementia tend to have more severe hearing loss. Some of the signs of hearing loss can mimic dementia. For example, individuals with hearing loss may misunderstand the auditory message and appear to be confused. If dementia is suspected, the audiologist can then conduct a screening of mental status using the Short Portable Mental Status Questionnaire (MSQ) (Pfeiffer, 1975). The audiological test battery may need to be modified. Some older adults with dementia may not be able to respond consistently to pure tone stimuli. Therefore, speech audiometry, in conjunction with objective assessments such as immittance testing, OAEs, and auditory-evoked potentials can provide valuable information about the status of the auditory system. Based on the test results, decisions will need to be made about the type(s) of amplification device to recommend. In this population it may be better to recommend an assistive listening device such as a PocketTalker or FM system rather than a hearing aid, to prevent the device from being lost.

In summary, as demographics of the U.S. population change to include more elderly, there is going to be a growing demand to offer hearing health care services to this diverse group. As baby boomers age, there will be more demand for high-quality technological amplification devices. In addition, more auditory rehabilitation services can be offered through the Internet, home-based programs, and telehealth services. More audiologists will spend the majority of their caseload with this population over the next several decades. It is imperative that audiologists have a thorough understanding of the multifaceted issues this complex population is facing as they age in a healthy and successful manner so that cost-effective, interdisciplinary hearing health care services can be provided.

AUDIOLOGIC REHABILITATION CONSIDERATIONS IN OLDER ADULTS

There are a variety of variables that need to be taken into account in designing effective auditory rehabilitations programs for older adults. The audiologic rehabilitation process for older adults is multifaceted due to the many biological, psychological, and social changes that accompany aging. Some of these factors include the following:

> *Visual status*—Adequate visual acuity is necessary to see the components of the amplification devices and to benefit from visual cues to supplement audition. The speed of visual processing is important to aid the speechreading process. Botwinick (1970) stated that with aging there may be slower processing of visual information. Whenever possible, low-vision devices (e.g., magnifiers) can be used to magnify the controls and print. Large-print materials should be used with older adults. (Busacco, 2009; Kriscos, 2008)

Auditory status—The older adult's peripheral and central auditory abilities are critical in determining the type of amplification devices to recommend. For example, if binaural interference is present, an older patient may benefit from one hearing aid and an FM listening system (Walden & Walden, 2005). When providing hearing health care services to older adults, a screening such as the QuickSin or HINT should be done routinely to determine whether accommodations need to be made possibly related to the presence of APD, which can impact significantly on speech perception abilities.

Manual dexterity—The elderly individual's manual dexterity needs to be assessed. The ability to insert, remove, and manipulate the controls of an amplification device is critical to its successful use. With aging, the decrease in touch sensitivity can impact the ability to adjust the controls of the hearing aid (Hull, 2004). It is recommended that remote controls and automatic controls be used with this population. If there are significant manual dexterity problems, a referral to an occupational therapist should be considered because hearing aid usage falls under the definition of an activity of daily living (ADL) (Busacco, 2009). The more independent an older adult is with the amplification device, the more likely that it will be used on a consistent basis.

Cognition—In order to benefit maximally from the audiological rehabilitation process, adequate cognition is necessary. One goal of the audiological rehabilitation program is to promote the use of the cognitive processes necessary to derive meaning from incomplete sensory messages. If there are significant cognitive deficits due to aging, it may be necessary to have a caretaker insert and remove the amplification device(s). The use of a hearing aid may improve cognitive functioning (Mulrow, Agular, Endicott, & Tulley, 1990). When conducting tests to assess cognitive functioning, some type of amplification device such as a PocketTalker should be used to ensure that the speech signal is audible so as to enhance speech understanding.

Psychological status—Assessment of the older adult's psychological status is critical to the success of an audiologic rehabilitation process. According to a study conducted by the National Council on Aging (1999), older adults with untreated hearing loss are more likely than their counterparts who use hearing aids to experience higher levels of depression, anger, and frustration. A successful auditory rehabilitation program will address the role of grief and mourning on the older person's acceptance of the hearing loss. If one does not accept the hearing loss, the motivational level to engage in audiologic rehabilitation will be affected. The higher the motivational level, the more successful the outcomes of the auditory rehabilitation program. Realistic expectations also are critical about the benefits of amplification. Unrealistic expectations will impact on the long-term benefits derived from the hearing rehabilitation process. In cases of depression and reduced quality of life despite auditory intervention, a referral to a psychological professional may be necessary (Trychin, 1995).

The involvement of the older adult's family is critical. If an older person is a nursing home resident, essential staff must be involved in the rehabilitation process. It is critical that the audiologic rehabilitation program be modified based on the changing biological, psychological, and social needs of the older patient. As one ages, there will be numerous age-related challenges that may change on a yearly basis. Regular follow-up will better ensure appropriate hearing health care services are provided to this growing population in the United States.

Audiogram Interpretation Exercises

PATIENT 1

Mr. J., an 82-year-old male, was seen for an initial audiological assessment. He is in a blind rehabilitation program due to macular degeneration. Over the course of the last three months, Mr. J. has stated that his vision loss has gotten progressively worse. He has worn in-the-ear hearing aids for 10 years. At this time the hearing aids are not working. Mr. J. is very concerned about his hearing loss, as he needs to depend on auditory cues for his activities of daily living (ADLs). He reported problems understanding speech in noise and also picking up on auditory cues when using his cane for mobility and orientation purposes. He has no family in the immediate geographical area. He stated that he hopes to get an aide to assist him on a 24-hour basis in his home. Mr. J. said that he is feeling very depressed about his combined vision and hearing loss. He attained a score of 22 on the HHIE, suggesting a moderate hearing handicap.

1. Describe the pure tone results in both ears. Calculate the three-frequency pure-tone average in each ear.

2. Describe the word recognition results in each ear.

3. Interpret the HHIE score. of 22.

4. What other professionals would you coordinate the audiological rehabilitation plan for Mr. J.?

5. What are two recommendations that you would make for Mr. J.?

NAME: Patient 1   AGE/DATE OF BIRTH: 82 y/o

REFERRED BY: _____   MEDICAL RECORD #: _____

TEST INTERVAL: _____   DATE OF TEST: _____

PURE TONE AUDIOMETRY (RE: ANSI 1996)

KEY:		
LEFT	STIMULUS	RIGHT
X	AIR	O
□	AIR - MASK	Δ
>	BONE	<
]	BONE - MASK	[
↘	NO RESPONSE	✓
L	AIDED SOUND FIELD	R
	SOUND FIELD = S	

TEST TYPE
- STANDARD CAE
- PLAY
- COR/VRA
- BOA

TRANSDUCER
- INSERT
- CIRCUMAURAL
- SOUND FIELD

RELIABILITY
- EXCELLENT
- GOOD
- FAIR
- POOR

BOOTH
- #1
- #2 (PEDS)
- #3
- #4 COCH IMPLANT

TYMPANOMETRY (226 Hz)

EAR	LEFT	RIGHT
STATIC ADMITTANCE (mm H₂O)		
TYMP PEAK PRESSURE (DaPa)		
TYMP WIDTH (DaPa)		
EAR CANAL VOLUME cm³		

LEFT   RIGHT

Admittance

Pressure   Pressure

CONTRA	.5k Hz	1k Hz	2k Hz	4k Hz	IPSI	.5k Hz	1k Hz	2k Hz	4k Hz
Right (AD) (phone ear)	95	95	100	105	AD (probe ear)	90	95	90	
Left (AS) (phone ear)	95	95	95		AS (probe ear)	90	90	90	

MIDDLE EAR ANALYZER _____

SPEECH AUDIOMETRY

	PTA	SRT/SAT	Speech Recognition		Speech Recognition		MCL	UCL
RIGHT (AD)	40		76 %	75	%		75	
Masking								
LEFT (AS)	45		80 %	75	%		75	
Masking								

MLV □	CD/tape ☒	W-22 □	WIPI □	PBK □	SPECIAL: NU- 6	SPECIAL:
SOUND FIELD		%		%		
RIGHT AIDED		%		%		
LEFT AIDED		%		%		
BINAURAL		%		%		

OTOACOUSTIC EMISSIONS (OAEs)

EMISSION TYPE USED	TEST TYPE PERFORMED
Transient	OAE Complete
Distortion Product	OAE Screening

OAE results:

Right Ear	Absent
Left Ear	Absent

OAE UNIT _____

HEARING AID INFORMATION

RIGHT AID: _____

LEFT AID: _____

OTOSCOPY: _____

HISTORY/IMPRESSIONS/RECOMMENDATIONS: _____

_____

_____

_____

_____

_____

AUDIOLOGIST: _____   ASSISTANT: _____   AUDIOMETER: _____

FIGURE 3.1   Patient 1

Audiogram Interpretation Exercises

PATIENT 2

Mrs. B., a 67-year-old woman, was seen for an audiological evaluation. She was accompanied to the evaluation by her husband of forty years. She reported experiencing a sudden hearing loss in her right ear accompanied by roaring tinnitus, nausea, and vertigo for the past three weeks. She also reported a hearing loss in her left ear. The vertigo has subsided over the past several days. Mrs. B. is very concerned that the vertigo will incapacitate her, she has not been able to drive or walk without feeling a tendency to fall. Mrs. B. reported that she has hypertension and takes medication on a daily basis. Otherwise, her general health is good.

1. Describe the pure tone results in each ear.

2. What would you expect the SRT to be in ear each based on the pure tone results?

3. Describe the word recognition results in each ear.

4. What can account for the difference in word recognition scores between the ears?

5. What do you think is the possible etiology of the hearing loss in each ear?

6. Why do you think there was positive acoustic reflex decay in the right ear at 1000 Hz at 10 dB SL?

7. What are three recommendations that you would make for this patient?

NAME: Patient 2   AGE/DATE OF BIRTH: 67 y/o

REFERRED BY: _____   MEDICAL RECORD #: _____

TEST INTERVAL: _____   DATE OF TEST: _____

PURE TONE AUDIOMETRY (RE: ANSI 1996)

KEY:

	STIMULUS	
LEFT		RIGHT
X	AIR	O
□	AIR - MASK	Δ
>	BONE	<
]	BONE - MASK	[
↘	NO RESPONSE	✓
L	AIDED SOUND FIELD	R
	SOUND FIELD = S	

TEST TYPE
- STANDARD CAE
- PLAY
- COR/VRA
- BOA

TRANSDUCER
- INSERT
- CIRCUMAURAL
- SOUND FIELD

RELIABILITY
- EXCELLENT
- GOOD
- FAIR
- POOR

BOOTH
- #1
- #2 (PEDS)
- #3
- #4 COCH IMPLANT

TYMPANOMETRY (226 Hz)

EAR	LEFT	RIGHT
STATIC ADMITTANCE (mm H$_2$O)		
TYMP PEAK PRESSURE (DaPa)		
TYMP WIDTH (DaPa)		
EAR CANAL VOLUME cm^3		

LEFT   Pressure

RIGHT   Pressure

CONTRA	5k Hz	1k Hz	2k Hz	4k Hz	IPSI	5k Hz	1k Hz	2k Hz	4k Hz
Right (AD) (phone ear)	100	100	100	100	AD (probe ear)	90	95	95	
Left (AS) (phone ear)	95	100	100		AS (probe ear)	90	95	100	

MIDDLE EAR ANALYZER _____

SPEECH AUDIOMETRY

	PTA	SRT/ SAT	Speech Recognition	Speech Recognition	MCL	UCL
RIGHT (AD)	50		72 % 90	%		
Masking			72 % 70			
LEFT (AS)	40		84 % 80	%		
Masking			84 % 60			

MLV □	CD/tape ☒	W-22 □	WIPI □	PBK □	SPECIAL: NU- 6	SPECIAL:
SOUND FIELD			%		%	
RIGHT AIDED			%		%	
LEFT AIDED			%		%	
BINAURAL			%		%	

OTOACOUSTIC EMISSIONS (OAEs)

EMISSION TYPE USED	TEST TYPE PERFORMED
Transient	OAE Complete
Distortion Product	OAE Screening
OAE results:	
Right Ear Present	
Left Ear Absent	

OAE UNIT _____

HEARING AID INFORMATION

RIGHT AID: _____

LEFT AID: _____

OTOSCOPY: _____

HISTORY/IMPRESSIONS/RECOMMENDATIONS: Acoustic Reflex Decay was positive in the right ear at 1000Hz. Acoustic reflex decay was negative at 500Hz in the right ear. Acoustic reflex decay was negative at 500HZ and 1000Hz in the left ear.

_____

_____

_____

_____

AUDIOLOGIST: _____   ASSISTANT: _____   AUDIOMETER: _____

FIGURE 3.2   Patient 2

Audiogram Interpretation Exercises

PATIENT 3

Dr. P., age 76, was seen for an annual audiological reevaluation. He has been a patient at the hearing and balance clinic for approximately five years. At present, he uses bilateral digital multimemory hearing aids. He purchased the hearing aids two years ago. Initially, he reported benefit using two hearing aids. At this time he is using only one hearing aid in his right ear. Dr. P. stated that he does not believe two hearing aids are helping him and he prefers to use one hearing aid. He reports that when wearing two hearing aids he has a great deal of difficulty understanding speech in the presence of background noise.

1. Describe the pure tone thresholds.

2. Describe binaural aided word recognition results as compared to monaural aided word recognition results. What does the difference between these test results suggest?

3. What can be the cause of the poor aided binaural word recognition score compared to the monaural aided conditions?

4. What are the implications of an auditory processing disorder for hearing aid fitting?

NAME: Patient 3 AGE/DATE OF BIRTH: 76 y/o

REFERRED BY: _____ MEDICAL RECORD #: _____

TEST INTERVAL: _____ DATE OF TEST: _____

PURE TONE AUDIOMETRY (RE: ANSI 1996)

KEY:

LEFT	STIMULUS	RIGHT
X	AIR	O
☐	AIR - MASK	Δ
>	BONE	<
]	BONE - MASK	[
↓	NO RESPONSE	↓
L	AIDED SOUND FIELD	R
	SOUND FIELD = S	

TEST TYPE
| STANDARD CAE |
| PLAY |
| COR/VRA |
| BOA |

TRANSDUCER
| INSERT |
| CIRCUMAURAL |
| SOUND FIELD |

RELIABILITY
| EXCELLENT |
| GOOD |
| FAIR |
| POOR |

BOOTH
| #1 |
| #2 (PEDS) |
| #3 |
| #4 COCH IMPLANT |

TYMPANOMETRY (226 Hz)

EAR	LEFT	RIGHT
STATIC ADMITTANCE (mm H₂O)		
TYMP PEAK PRESSURE (DaPa)		
TYMP WIDTH (DaPa)		
EAR CANAL VOLUME cm³		

CONTRA	5k Hz	1k Hz	2k Hz	4k Hz	IPSI	5k Hz	1k Hz	2k Hz	4k Hz
Right (AD) (phone ear)					AD (probe ear)				
Left (AS) (phone ear)					AS (probe ear)				

MIDDLE EAR ANALYZER _____

SPEECH AUDIOMETRY

	PTA	SRT/SAT	Speech Recognition		Speech Recognition		MCL	UCL
RIGHT (AD)	60		56 %	90	%			
Masking								
LEFT (AS)	60		50 %	90	%			
Masking								

MLV ☐	CD/tape ☒	W-22 ☒	WIPI ☐	PBK ☐	SPECIAL:		SPECIAL:
SOUND FIELD			%		%		
RIGHT AIDED			54 %		%		
LEFT AIDED			46 %		%		
BINAURAL			36 %		%		

OTOACOUSTIC EMISSIONS (OAEs)

EMISSION TYPE USED	TEST TYPE PERFORMED
Transient	OAE Complete
Distortion Product	OAE Screening
OAE results:	
Right Ear	
Left Ear	

OAE UNIT _____

HEARING AID INFORMATION

RIGHT AID: _____

LEFT AID: _____

OTOSCOPY: _____

HISTORY/IMPRESSIONS/RECOMMENDATIONS: _____

_____

_____

_____

_____

_____

AUDIOLOGIST: _____ ASSISTANT: _____ AUDIOMETER: _____

FIGURE 3.3 Patient 3

PATIENT 4

Mr. S., age 88, is a resident of a long-term care facility. He has been at the nursing home facility for three years. The staff at the nursing home is concerned about Mr. S's. hearing because oftentimes he answers inappropriately and appears to be confused. The staff does not know whether his confusion is the result of a hearing loss, cognitive deficits, or both.

Mr. S. was placed in the nursing home because he cannot live independently due to mobility issues and lack of family support for caregiving. When questioned by the audiologist, Mr. S. stated that he does not understand the staff at the facility. Everyone appears to "mumble." He feels isolated and depressed. He cannot participate in recreational activities due to his inability to follow directions and understand speech, especially of other residents. The HHIE-N (i.e., Nursing Home Version) yielded a score of 40 and the HHIE–Staff Version yielded a score of 32, suggesting a significant hearing handicap.

1. Why do you think that there are no pure tone test results for Mr. S.?

2. Describe the word recognition results in each ear.

3. Describe the OAE results.

4. Describe the immittance results.

5. What are the results of the HHIE-N version for the resident and the HHIE Staff Version?

6. Interpret the results of the audiological test battery to determine the type and degree of hearing loss.

7. What audiologic recommendations should be made for this patient?

NAME: Patient 4 **AGE/DATE OF BIRTH:** 88 y/o

REFERRED BY: _____ **MEDICAL RECORD #:** _____

TEST INTERVAL: _____ **DATE OF TEST:** _____

PURE TONE AUDIOMETRY (RE: ANSI 1996)

KEY:

LEFT	Stimulus	RIGHT
X	AIR	O
☐	AIR - MASK	△
>	BONE	<
]	BONE - MASK	[
↘	NO RESPONSE	✓
L	AIDED SOUND FIELD	R

SOUND FIELD = S

TEST TYPE
- STANDARD/CAE
- PLAY
- COR/VRA
- BOA

TRANSDUCER
- INSERT
- CIRCUMAURAL
- SOUND FIELD

RELIABILITY
- EXCELLENT
- GOOD
- FAIR
- POOR

BOOTH
- #1
- #2 (PEDS)
- #3
- #4 COCH IMPLANT

TYMPANOMETRY (226 Hz)

EAR	LEFT	RIGHT
STATIC ADMITTANCE (mm H$_2$O)		
TYMP PEAK PRESSURE (DaPa)		
TYMP WIDTH (DaPa)		
EAR CANAL VOLUME cm^3		

LEFT — Pressure | RIGHT — Pressure

CONTRA	5k Hz	1k Hz	2k Hz	4k Hz	IPSI	5k Hz	1k Hz	2k Hz	4k Hz
Right (AD) (phone ear)					AD (probe ear)				
Left (AS) (phone ear)					AS (probe ear)				

NR | NR

MIDDLE EAR ANALYZER _____

SPEECH AUDIOMETRY

	PTA	SRT/SAT	Speech Recognition		Speech Recognition		MCL	UCL
RIGHT (AD)		70	64%	95	%			
Masking								
LEFT (AS)		75	64%	95	%			
Masking								

MLV ☒	CD/tape ☐	W-22 ☒	WIPI ☐	PBK ☐	SPECIAL:	SPECIAL:	
SOUND FIELD			%		%		
RIGHT AIDED			%		%		
LEFT AIDED			%		%		
BINAURAL			%		%		

OTOACOUSTIC EMISSIONS (OAEs)

EMISSION TYPE USED	TEST TYPE PERFORMED
Transient	OAE Complete
Distortion Product	OAE Screening
OAE results:	
Right Ear Absent	
Left Ear Absent	

OAE UNIT _____

HEARING AID INFORMATION

RIGHT AID: _____

LEFT AID: _____

OTOSCOPY: _____

HISTORY/IMPRESSIONS/RECOMMENDATIONS: Could not test pure tones. _____

_____

_____

_____

_____

_____

AUDIOLOGIST: _____ **ASSISTANT:** _____ **AUDIOMETER:** _____

FIGURE 3.4 Patient 4

PATIENT 5:

Mrs. Q. age 75, was seen for an initial audiological evaluation. She stated that she is seen twice a year by an ENT physician to remove excessive cerumen. Her last visit was about five months ago. Otoscopic examination revealed clear ear canals bilaterally, with stenosis of the ear canals noted by the audiologist. Her pinnae were extremely flaccid. She reported no significant hearing loss that interferes with her ability to communicate in a variety of listening environments. Her case history revealed no significant medical disorders. She does not take any medications on a regular basis.

1. In reviewing all of the presented audiological data, what concerns you about the data? Are here any inconsistencies present in the data?

2. What could be the reasons for the air-bone gaps at 2000 Hz and 4000 Hz in each ear?

3. What procedure can be used to eliminate collapsed canals?

4. Describe the immittance results in each ear.

5. Describe the OAE results in each ear.

6. What recommendation would you make for Mrs. Q.?

NAME: Patient 5   AGE/DATE OF BIRTH: 75 y/o

REFERRED BY: _____   MEDICAL RECORD #: _____

TEST INTERVAL: _____   DATE OF TEST: _____

PURE TONE AUDIOMETRY (RE: ANSI 1996)

KEY:

	LEFT Stimulus RIGHT	
X	AIR	O
□	AIR - MASK	Δ
>	BONE	<
]	BONE - MASK	[
↘	NO RESPONSE	✓
L	AIDED SOUND FIELD	R
	SOUND FIELD = S	

TEST TYPE
- STANDARD CAE
- PLAY
- COR/VRA
- BOA

TRANSDUCER
- INSERT
- CIRCUMAURAL
- SOUND FIELD

RELIABILITY
- EXCELLENT
- GOOD
- FAIR
- POOR

BOOTH
- #1
- #2 (PEDS)
- #3
- #4 COCH IMPLANT

TYMPANOMETRY (226 Hz)

EAR	LEFT	RIGHT
STATIC ADMITTANCE (mm H₂O)		
TYMP PEAK PRESSURE (DaPa)		
TYMP WIDTH (DaPa)		
EAR CANAL VOLUME cm³		

LEFT   RIGHT

Admittance

Pressure   Pressure

CONTRA	.5k Hz	1k Hz	2k Hz	4k Hz	IPSI	.5k Hz	1k Hz	2k Hz	4k Hz
Right (AD) (phone ear)	95	90	95	100	AD (probe ear)	95	90	95	
Left (AS) (phone ear)	95	95	95	95	AS (probe ear)	95	95	95	

MIDDLE EAR ANALYZER _____

SPEECH AUDIOMETRY

	PTA	SRT/SAT	Speech Recognition	Speech Recognition	MCL	UCL
RIGHT (AD)			%	%		
Masking						
LEFT (AS)			%	%		
Masking						

MLV □	CD/tape □	W-22 □	WIPI □	PBK □	SPECIAL:	SPECIAL:
SOUND FIELD			%		%	
RIGHT AIDED			%		%	
LEFT AIDED			%		%	
BINAURAL			%		%	

OTOACOUSTIC EMISSIONS (OAEs)

EMISSION TYPE USED	TEST TYPE PERFORMED
Transient	OAE Complete
Distortion Product	OAE Screening
OAE results:	
Right Ear	Present
Left Ear	Present

OAE UNIT _____

HEARING AID INFORMATION

RIGHT AID: _____

LEFT AID: _____

OTOSCOPY: _____

HISTORY/IMPRESSIONS/RECOMMENDATIONS: _____

_____

_____

_____

_____

_____

AUDIOLOGIST: _____   ASSISTANT: _____   AUDIOMETER: _____

FIGURE 3.5 Patient 5

Audiogram Interpretation Exercises

PATIENT 6

Mrs. F., age 74, has been a long-time audiology patient. She suffered a sudden bilateral severe-to-profound sensorineural hearing loss about two years ago. Despite numerous medical evaluations, the etiology of the hearing loss could not be obtained. Mrs. F. has been using bilateral power behind-the-ear digital hearing aids. She reports limited benefit from the hearing aids. Mrs. F. is a retired school teacher. She is very active in community activities. At present, her daughter reports that Mrs. B. is becoming isolated and withdrawn due to her hearing loss. Mrs. F. is cognitively alert and in good physical health.

1. Describe the hearing test results.

2. Why was speech recognition testing not done?

3. In what types of situations do you think the patient has communication problems?

4. What are three recommendations you would make for this patient?

NAME: _Patient 6_

AGE/DATE OF BIRTH: ___74 y/o___

REFERRED BY: _____

MEDICAL RECORD #: _____

TEST INTERVAL: _____

DATE OF TEST: _____

PURE TONE AUDIOMETRY (RE: ANSI 1996)

KEY:

LEFT	STIMULUS	RIGHT
X	AIR	O
□	AIR - MASK	△
>	BONE	<
]	BONE - MASK	[
↘	NO RESPONSE	↙
L	AIDED SOUND FIELD	R
	SOUND FIELD = S	

TEST TYPE
STANDARD CAE
PLAY
COR/VRA
BOA

TRANSDUCER
INSERT
CIRCUMAURAL
SOUND FIELD

RELIABILITY
EXCELLENT
GOOD
FAIR
POOR

BOOTH
#1
#2 (PEDS)
#3
#4 COCH IMPLANT

TYMPANOMETRY (226 Hz)

EAR	LEFT	RIGHT
STATIC ADMITTANCE (mm H$_2$O)		
TYMP PEAK PRESSURE (DaPa)		
TYMP WIDTH (DaPa)		
EAR CANAL VOLUME cm^3		

LEFT — Pressure

RIGHT — Pressure

CONTRA	.5k Hz	1k Hz	2k Hz	4k Hz	IPSI	.5k Hz	1k Hz	2k Hz	4k Hz
Right (AD) (phone ear)		NR			AD (probe ear)		NR		
Left (AS) (phone ear)					AS (probe ear)				

MIDDLE EAR ANALYZER _____

SPEECH AUDIOMETRY

	PTA	SRT/SAT	Speech Recognition	Speech Recognition	MCL	UCL
RIGHT (AD)	85	CNT %		%		
Masking						
LEFT (AS)	85	CNT %		%		
Masking						

MLV ☒	CD/tape □	W-22 □	WIPI □	PBK □	SPECIAL:	SPECIAL:
SOUND FIELD					%	%
RIGHT AIDED					%	%
LEFT AIDED					%	%
BINAURAL					%	%

OTOACOUSTIC EMISSIONS (OAEs)

EMISSION TYPE USED	TEST TYPE PERFORMED
Transient	OAE Complete
Distortion Product	OAE Screening
OAE results:	
Right Ear	
Left Ear	

OAE UNIT _____

HEARING AID INFORMATION

RIGHT AID: _____

LEFT AID: _____

OTOSCOPY: _____

HISTORY/IMPRESSIONS/RECOMMENDATIONS: _____

_____

_____

_____

_____

_____

AUDIOLOGIST: _____   ASSISTANT: _____   AUDIOMETER: _____

FIGURE 3.6 Patient 6

PATIENT 7

Dr. O., age 65, was seen for an audiological evaluation and hearing aid check. She was seen at this clinic three years ago. At that time, she was fitted monaurally in the right ear with a digital mini behind-the-ear hearing aid. She refused to use a hearing aid in the left ear despite being a good candidate for binaural amplification. Audiologic results at that time revealed a mild to moderately severe, gradually sloping sensorineural hearing loss bilaterally. Word recognition results were 88% bilaterally at 35 dB SL re: SRT. Immittance results suggested normal middle-ear functioning bilaterally.

1. Describe the audiological results in both ears that were obtained three years ago in Audiogram 1 as compared to current audiological data depicted in Audiogram 2.

2. What might account for the decrease in word recognition results in the left ear as compared to the right ear?

3. What recommendations would you make?

NAME: Patient 7-A

REFERRED BY: _____

TEST INTERVAL: _____

AGE/DATE OF BIRTH: 65 y/o

MEDICAL RECORD #: _____

DATE OF TEST: _____

PURE TONE AUDIOMETRY (RE: ANSI 1996)

KEY:

LEFT	STIMULUS	RIGHT
X	AIR	O
☐	AIR - MASK	△
>	BONE	<
]	BONE - MASK	[
↘	NO RESPONSE	✓
L	AIDED SOUND FIELD	R
	SOUND FIELD = S	

TEST TYPE
STANDARD CAE
PLAY
COR/VRA
BOA

TRANSDUCER
INSERT
CIRCUMAURAL
SOUND FIELD

RELIABILITY
EXCELLENT
GOOD
FAIR
POOR

BOOTH
#1
#2 (PEDS)
#3
#4 COCH IMPLANT

TYMPANOMETRY (226 Hz)

EAR	LEFT	RIGHT
STATIC ADMITTANCE (mm H₂O)		
TYMP PEAK PRESSURE (DaPa)		
TYMP WIDTH (DaPa)		
EAR CANAL VOLUME cm³		

LEFT

RIGHT

Pressure

Pressure

CONTRA	5k Hz	1k Hz	2k Hz	4k Hz	IPSI	5k Hz	1k Hz	2k Hz	4k Hz
Right (AD) (phone ear)	85	85	90	100	AD (probe ear)	85	85	90	
Left (AS) (phone ear)	90	90	90	100	AS (probe ear)	95	95	90	

MIDDLE EAR ANALYZER _____

SPEECH AUDIOMETRY

	PTA	SRT/SAT	Speech Recognition		Speech Recognition		MCL	UCL
RIGHT (AD)	50	55	88%	90	88%	90		
Masking								
LEFT (AS)	50	55	88%	90	60%	90		
Masking								

MLV ☐	CD/tape ☒	W-22 ☐	WIPI ☐	PBK ☐	SPECIAL: NU-6	SPECIAL:
SOUND FIELD		%		%		
RIGHT AIDED		%		%		
LEFT AIDED		%		%		
BINAURAL		%		%		

OTOACOUSTIC EMISSIONS (OAEs)

EMISSION TYPE USED	TEST TYPE PERFORMED
Transient	OAE Complete
Distortion Product	OAE Screening
OAE results:	
Right Ear	
Left Ear	

OAE UNIT _____

HEARING AID INFORMATION

RIGHT AID: _____

LEFT AID: _____

OTOSCOPY: _____

HISTORY/IMPRESSIONS/RECOMMENDATIONS: _____

_____

_____

_____

_____

AUDIOLOGIST: _____ ASSISTANT: _____ AUDIOMETER: _____

FIGURE 3.7A Patient 7, Audiogram 1

NAME: Patient 7-B AGE/DATE OF BIRTH: 65 y/o

REFERRED BY: _____ MEDICAL RECORD #: _____

TEST INTERVAL: _____ DATE OF TEST: _____

PURE TONE AUDIOMETRY (RE: ANSI 1996)

KEY:

LEFT	STIMULUS	RIGHT
X	AIR	O
☐	AIR - MASK	Δ
>	BONE	<
]	BONE - MASK	[
↘	NO RESPONSE	✓
L	AIDED SOUND FIELD	R
	SOUND FIELD = S	

TEST TYPE

STANDARD OAE	
PLAY	
COR/VRA	
BOA	

TRANSDUCER

INSERT	
CIRCUMAURAL	
SOUND FIELD	

RELIABILITY

EXCELLENT	
GOOD	
FAIR	
POOR	

BOOTH

#1	
#2 (PEDS)	
#3	
#4 COCH IMPLANT	

TYMPANOMETRY (226 Hz)

EAR	LEFT	RIGHT
STATIC ADMITTANCE (mm H₂O)		
TYMP PEAK PRESSURE (DaPa)		
TYMP WIDTH (DaPa)		
EAR CANAL VOLUME cm³		

LEFT   RIGHT
Pressure   Pressure

CONTRA	5k Hz	1k Hz	2k Hz	4k Hz	IPSI	5k Hz	1k Hz	2k Hz	4k Hz
Right (AD) (phone ear)	85	85	90	100	AD (probe ear)	85	85	90	
Left (AS) (phone ear)	90	90	90	100	AS (probe ear)	95	95	90	

MIDDLE EAR ANALYZER _____

SPEECH AUDIOMETRY

	PTA	SRT/SAT	Speech Recognition	Speech Recognition	MCL	UCL
RIGHT (AD)	50	55	88%	90	%	
Masking						
LEFT (AS)	50	55	60%	90	%	
Masking						

MLV ☐	CD/tape ☒	W-22 ☐	WIPI ☐	PBK ☐	SPECIAL: NU- 6	SPECIAL:
SOUND FIELD		%		%		
RIGHT AIDED		%		%		
LEFT AIDED		%		%		
BINAURAL		%		%		

OTOACOUSTIC EMISSIONS (OAEs)

EMISSION TYPE USED	TEST TYPE PERFORMED
Transient	OAE Complete
Distortion Product	OAE Screening
OAE results:	
Right Ear	
Left Ear	

OAE UNIT _____

HEARING AID INFORMATION

RIGHT AID: _____

LEFT AID: _____

OTOSCOPY: _____

HISTORY/IMPRESSIONS/RECOMMENDATIONS: _____

_____

_____

_____

_____

_____

AUDIOLOGIST: _____ ASSISTANT: _____ AUDIOMETER: _____

FIGURE 3.7B Patient 7, Audiogram 2

J.S., age 85, resides in a long-term care facility for the past six months. He was referred to the facility because of some changes in cognitive status over the last year. His family has reported that he appears confused and disoriented. This has resulted in an inability to maintain independent living skills. His wife of 55 years died last year. J.S. has a history of hearing loss but has refused audiological intervention. The nursing home staff is very concerned that J.S.'s hearing loss is causing severe depression. He does not participate in any activities at the nursing home due to his poor communication skills. His family is very concerned about his mental status, communication skills, and depression. J.S. states that the does not care about his hearing loss because there is "no one" to talk to since his wife has died and his relocation to the nursing home. J.S. does not want a hearing aid because he is "too old" and does not want to spend the money since he "will die soon."

1. Describe the audiological test results obtained on J.S.

2. Why do you think J.S. could not participate in pure tone testing?

3. What additional objective assessments should be done to obtain more information about hearing status?

4. What amplification recommendations would you make based on hearing loss and cognitive status?

5. Describe the components of an in-service program that you would conduct for the staff at the nursing home. The in-service program should address the specific needs of J.S.

NAME: Patient 8   AGE/DATE OF BIRTH: 85 y/o
REFERRED BY: _____   MEDICAL RECORD #: _____
TEST INTERVAL: _____   DATE OF TEST: _____

PURE TONE AUDIOMETRY (RE: ANSI 1996)

CNT

TYMPANOMETRY (226 Hz)

EAR	LEFT	RIGHT
STATIC ADMITTANCE (mm H$_2$O)		
TYMP PEAK PRESSURE (DaPa)		
TYMP WIDTH (DaPa)		
EAR CANAL VOLUME cm^3		

LEFT — Pressure / Admittance / RIGHT — Pressure

CONTRA	.5k Hz	1k Hz	2k Hz	4k Hz	IPSI	.5k Hz	1k Hz	2k Hz	4k Hz
Right (AD) (phone ear)	90	90	95	NR	AD (probe ear)	80	85	90	
Left (AS) (phone ear)	90	90	85	NR	AS (probe ear)	85	90	95	

MIDDLE EAR ANALYZER _____

SPEECH AUDIOMETRY

	PTA	SRT/SAT	Speech Recognition		Speech Recognition		MCL	UCL
RIGHT (AD)	35		72 %	75 40dB$L	%			
Masking								
LEFT (AS)	45		76 %	85 40dB$L	%			
Masking								

MLV ☒	CD/tape ☐	W-22 ☒	WIPI ☐	PBK ☐	SPECIAL:	SPECIAL:
SOUND FIELD			%		%	
RIGHT AIDED			%		%	
LEFT AIDED			%		%	
BINAURAL			%		%	

OTOACOUSTIC EMISSIONS (OAEs)

EMISSION TYPE USED	TEST TYPE PERFORMED
Transient	OAE Complete
Distortion Product	OAE Screening
OAE results:	
Right Ear	
Left Ear	

OAE UNIT _____

HEARING AID INFORMATION

RIGHT AID: _____
LEFT AID: _____
OTOSCOPY: _____

HISTORY/IMPRESSIONS/RECOMMENDATIONS: Acoustic reflex decay was negative bilaterally at 500Hz and 1000Hz.

AUDIOLOGIST: _____   ASSISTANT: _____   AUDIOMETER: _____

FIGURE 3.8 Patient 8

PART 3 Audiological Diagnosis and Management of Hearing Loss in the Older Adult Population

PATIENT 9

Mr. A., age 60, was seen for an audiological evaluation. Mr. A. was diagnosed with Lyme disease one year ago. An avid hunter, Mr. A. was bitten by a tick about five years ago. He was treated with large doses of antibiotics after the tick bite was evidenced. Mr. A. has severe problems walking as a result of advanced Lyme disease. Over the last year, his mobility has deteriorated. He experiences bouts of dizziness that at times can be incapacitating. At present, Mr. A. uses a walker to get around. He appears confused, which is a common symptom associated with advanced Lyme disease. His family has noticed hearing difficulties. He also reported high-pitched tinnitus in both ears that interferes with his activities of daily living (ADLs). The tinnitus interferes with sleeping and is very bothersome in quiet environments. He appears to be depressed and withdrawn. He spends the majority of his time alone. His wife is very concerned about his lack of communication with family and friends and withdrawal from activities that were once enjoyable.

1. What type of hearing loss is usually associated with advanced Lyme disease?

2. Draw an audiogram that depicts that following:
   Moderate-to-profound sensorineural hearing loss
   Normal middle ear functioning bilaterally
   Fair word recognition ability at 40 dB SL re: SRT

3. Fill in the acoustic reflex data you would expect based on the pure tone results in each ear.

4. What audiologic management decision would you make?

NAME: Patient 9   AGE/DATE OF BIRTH: 60 y/o

REFERRED BY: _____   MEDICAL RECORD #: _____

TEST INTERVAL: _____   DATE OF TEST: _____

PURE TONE AUDIOMETRY (RE: ANSI 1996)

KEY:		
LEFT	STIMULUS	RIGHT
X	AIR	O
☐	AIR - MASK	Δ
>	BONE	<
]	BONE - MASK	[
↘	NO RESPONSE	✓
L	AIDED SOUND FIELD	R
	SOUND FIELD = S	

TEST TYPE
- STANDARD CAE
- PLAY
- COR/VRA
- BOA

TRANSDUCER
- INSERT
- CIRCUMAURAL
- SOUND FIELD

RELIABILITY
- EXCELLENT
- GOOD
- FAIR
- POOR

BOOTH
- #1
- #2 (PEDS)
- #3
- #4 COCH IMPLANT

TYMPANOMETRY (226 Hz)

EAR	LEFT	RIGHT
STATIC ADMITTANCE (mm H₂O)		
TYMP PEAK PRESSURE (DaPa)		
TYMP WIDTH (DaPa)		
EAR CANAL VOLUME cm³		

LEFT   Admittance   RIGHT

Pressure   Pressure

CONTRA	5k Hz	1k Hz	2k Hz	4k Hz	IPSI	5k Hz	1k Hz	2k Hz	4k Hz
Right (AD) (phone ear)					AD (probe ear)				
Left (AS) (phone ear)					AS (probe ear)				

MIDDLE EAR ANALYZER _____

SPEECH AUDIOMETRY

	PTA	SRT/ SAT	Speech Recognition	Speech Recognition	MCL	UCL
RIGHT (AD)			%	%		
Masking						
LEFT (AS)			%	%		
Masking						

MLV ☐	CD/tape ☐	W-22 ☐	WIPI ☐	PBK ☐	SPECIAL:	SPECIAL:
SOUND FIELD		%	%		
RIGHT AIDED		%	%		
LEFT AIDED		%	%		
BINAURAL		%	%		

OTOACOUSTIC EMISSIONS (OAEs)

EMISSION TYPE USED	TEST TYPE PERFORMED
Transient	OAE Complete
Distortion Product	OAE Screening
OAE results:	
Right Ear	
Left Ear	

OAE UNIT _____

HEARING AID INFORMATION

RIGHT AID: _____

LEFT AID: _____

OTOSCOPY: _____

HISTORY/IMPRESSIONS/RECOMMENDATIONS: _____

_____

_____

_____

_____

_____

AUDIOLOGIST: _____   ASSISTANT: _____   AUDIOMETER: _____

FIGURE 3.9 Patient 9

PATIENT 10

L.M., an active 80-year-old female, was seen for an audiological evaluation. She was referred by her neurologist. She reported feeling dizzy and unsteady on her feet. L.M. reported a high-pitched tinnitus in her right ear that is constant. She also experiences a feeling of fullness or pressure in her right ear. She did not report any difficulty hearing in her left ear. L.M. takes medication for high blood pressure, high cholesterol, and diabetes. She was diagnosed with Type II diabetes about six years ago. She maintains good glucose control overall.

1. What concerns do you have about this patient's case history and audiogram?

2. What is the possible etiology of the hearing loss?

3. What recommendations should be made for this patient?

NAME: Patient 10   AGE/DATE OF BIRTH: 80 y/o

REFERRED BY: _____   MEDICAL RECORD #: _____

TEST INTERVAL: _____   DATE OF TEST: _____

PURE TONE AUDIOMETRY (RE: ANSI 1996)

KEY:

LEFT	Stimulus	Right
X	AIR	O
☐	AIR - MASK	Δ
>	BONE	<
]	BONE - MASK	[
↙	NO RESPONSE	✓
L	AIDED SOUND FIELD	R
	SOUND FIELD = S	

TEST TYPE
- STANDARD CAE
- PLAY
- COR/VRA
- BOA

TRANSDUCER
- INSERT
- CIRCUMAURAL
- SOUND FIELD

RELIABILITY
- EXCELLENT
- GOOD
- FAIR
- POOR

BOOTH
- #1
- #2 (PEDS)
- #3
- #4 COCH IMPLANT

TYMPANOMETRY (226 Hz)

EAR	LEFT	RIGHT
STATIC ADMITTANCE (mm H_2O)		
TYMP PEAK PRESSURE (DaPa)		
TYMP WIDTH (DaPa)		
EAR CANAL VOLUME cm^3		

LEFT   RIGHT
Pressure   Pressure

CONTRA	.5k Hz	1k Hz	2k Hz	4k Hz	IPSI	.5k Hz	1k Hz	2k Hz	4k Hz
Right (AD) (phone ear)		NR			AD (probe ear)		NR		
Left (AS) (phone ear)					AS (probe ear)				

MIDDLE EAR ANALYZER _____

SPEECH AUDIOMETRY

	PTA	SRT/ SAT	Speech Recognition	Speech Recognition	MCL	UCL
RIGHT (AD)	50		72 %	90	%	
Masking						
LEFT (AS)	CNT		CNT %		%	
Masking						

MLV ☐	CD/tape ☒	W-22 ☒	WIPI ☐	PBK ☐	SPECIAL:	SPECIAL:
SOUND FIELD			%		%	
RIGHT AIDED			%		%	
LEFT AIDED			%		%	
BINAURAL			%		%	

OTOACOUSTIC EMISSIONS (OAEs)

EMISSION TYPE USED	TEST TYPE PERFORMED
Transient	OAE Complete
Distortion Product	OAE Screening
OAE results:	
Right Ear	
Left Ear	

OAE UNIT _____

HEARING AID INFORMATION

RIGHT AID: _____

LEFT AID: _____

OTOSCOPY: _____

HISTORY/IMPRESSIONS/RECOMMENDATIONS: _____

_____

_____

_____

_____

_____

AUDIOLOGIST: _____   ASSISTANT: _____   AUDIOMETER: _____

FIGURE 3.10   Patient 10

PART 3   Audiological Diagnosis and Management of Hearing Loss in the Older Adult Population

Clinical Enrichment Projects

1. Research the incidence of auditory processing disorders in older adults. What are the audiologic implications of auditory processing disorders on the audiologic rehabilitation process? What are some auditory rehabilitation recommendations that you would make for elderly adults with peripheral hearing loss and an auditory processing disorder?

2. Research two hearing handicap scales that have been developed specifically for older adults. Address the reliability and validity of each scale. How would you incorporate the use of hearing handicap scales into your clinical practice with older adults?

3. What are some of the hearing health care issues that are predominant in providing services to nursing home residents?

4. Research adult-onset auditory deprivation. Based on this phenomena provide a rationale for the use of two hearing aids when feasible versus one hearing aid in adults and the elderly.

5. What testing protocol would you use to evaluate an 80-year-old woman with hearing loss and mild dementia who resides in the community? Provide a rationale for each test selected as part of the protocol.

6. Conduct research on the impact of aging on temporally altered speech (e.g., time-compressed speech, gap detection, reverberation). What are the implications of the research findings for the audiologic management of older adults?

7. Discuss the relationship between hearing loss, depression, and quality-of-life issues in the elderly.

Answers to Audiogram Interpretation Exercises

PATIENT 1

1. *Pure tone thresholds suggest a moderate flat sensorineural hearing loss in both ears. The three-frequency pure tone average is 40 dB HL in the right ear and 50 dB HL in the left ear.*
2. *The word recognition results are 76% in the right ear and 80% in the left ear when presented at the patient's MCL, suggesting fair word recognition abilities.*
3. *A score of 22 suggests a mild-to-moderate hearing handicap. Based on the results of the HHIE as well as Mr. J's. reporting of concern about his hearing loss, he is an excellent candidate for audiological rehabilitation.*
4. *Given that Mr. J. is currently enrolled in a rehabilitation program at the blind center, it is critical to work with the low-vision staff in implementing the audiolgical program. The patient's dual sensory loss needs to be addressed by both vision and hearing specialists.*
5. • *Bilateral behind-the-ear hearing aids with direct audio input for use with an assistive listening device such as an FM system or infrared system.*
   • *Possible use of personal vibratory device to be aware of auditory signals in the home environment such as the doorbell, telephone, alarm clock, or microwave.*

PATIENT 2

1. *Pure tone thresholds in the right ear suggest a moderately severe sensorineural hearing loss at 250–750 Hz rising to a moderate sensorineural hearing loss at 1000–8000 Hz. Pure tone results in the left ear suggest a mild to moderate*

sensorineural hearing loss. The three-frequency pure tone average is 50 dB HL in the right ear and 40 dB HL in the left ear.
2. *The SRT in the right ear should be between 45 dB HL and 55 dB HL and the left ear, 35–45 dB HL.*
3. *The score of 72% in the right ear is fair and the result of 84% in the left ear is good.*
4. *The difference in understanding speech in each ear is probably attributed to the poorer hearing sensitivity in the right ear in the low frequencies.*
5. *Ménière's disease is possible for the right ear based on the symptoms of fluctuating hearing loss, vertigo, nausea, and tinnitus. The hearing loss in the left ear is consistent with presbycusis.*
6. *Sometimes in the presence of Ménière's disease there will be positive acoustic reflex decay after 5 seconds. Typically, if the presentation level is increased, then there will not be acoustic reflex decay.*
7. • *Follow-up with ENT physician with specialization in Ménière's disease.*
   • *Balance evaluation.*
   • *Programmable digital hearing aids.*
   • *Support group for Ménière's disease.*
   • *Audiological reevaluation to motion hearing sensitivity.*

PATIENT 3

1. *Pure tone thresholds revealed a moderately severe flat sensorineural hearing loss bilaterally. Word recognition results presented at 40 dB SL re: SRT were 56% in the right ear and 50% in the left ear, suggesting significant difficulty understanding speech in quiet at a loud level.*

2. *Binaural aided word recognition was 36%. Monaural aided for the right ear was 54% and monaural aided for the left ear is 46%.*
3. *The most probable cause for the poor performance is binaural integration deficit (i.e., auditory processing disorders), which is common in the elderly population.*
4. *Oftentimes, older adults with both peripheral and central auditory involvement will benefit more from monaural than bilateral hearing aids. In addition, an assistive listening device such as an FM system should be considered to improve the signal-to-noise ratio and word recognition abilities.*

PATIENT 4

1. *It may be that he could not follow the directions for pure tone testing as a result of either the severity of hearing loss and/or some cognitive deficits.*
2. *The word recognition results of 64% in each ear suggest that Mr. S. has a great deal of difficulty understanding speech at loud levels in quiet.*
3. *DPOAE were not present in either ear, suggesting at least a moderate hearing loss since these are usually present in normal hearing and in mild hearing loss.*
4. *Tympanograms suggest normal middle-ear functioning. Contralateral and ipsilateral acoustic reflexes were not present at each frequency bilaterally, which is probably due to the severity of hearing loss.*
5. *Mr. S.'s HHIE score was 40, suggesting a significant hearing handicap. The HHIE was given to the nursing home staff to assess the staff's perception of the resident's hearing handicap. Their score was 32, which suggests significant hearing handicap exhibited by the resident as perceived by the staff of the facility.*
6. *Based on the composite of the test data, it appears that Mr. S. has a sensorineural hearing loss bilaterally. The degree of hearing loss is severe in both ears. He also reports that the hearing loss is impacting his lifestyle and quality of life. The severity of the untreated hearing loss may be causing confusion and disorientation.*
7. *Mr. S. is a hearing aid candidate for BTE aids. If he does not want hearing aids, then a hard-wired listening system would be appropriate. Staff in-service training is critical for successful*

amplification for this resident. It is uncertain at this time whether he can be an independent hearing aid user. It is recommended that Mr. S. be seen by an occupational therapist for assistance with hearing aid insertion and removal as an ADL.

PATIENT 5

1. *One inconsistency is the presence of air-bone gaps at 2000 Hz and 4000 Hz bilaterally. The presence of a conductive component is not consistent with immitance results, which suggests normal middle-ear function.*
2. *Conducting otoscopic examination, the ear canals were stenotic and the pinnae were extremely floppy, which can result in collapsing of the ear canal.*
3. *Use of insert earphones to eliminate the pressure caused by the TDH-49 earphones.*
4. *The immittance results in each ear suggest normal middle ear functioning. These results eliminate the possibility of a conductive or mixed hearing loss as suggested by the air-bone gaps at 2000–4000 Hz bilaterally. The presence of air-bone gaps may be erroneous due to of collapsed ear canals.*
5. *DPOAEs are present bilaterally, suggesting no conductive pathology.*
6. *Reevaluate using insert earphones.*

PATIENT 6

1. *Severe-to-profound sensorineural hearing loss bilaterally. Etiology remains unknown.*
2. *It was not done due to the severity of the hearing loss and the equipment output limitations for speech.*
3. *All communication situations would be problematic for this patient.*
4. • *Cochlear implant evaluation.*
   • *Use of assistive listening device(s).*
   • *Communication strategies training to improve functional communication skills.*

PATIENT 7

1. *Pure tone thresholds in both ears were consistent with mild to moderately severe, gradually sloping sensorineural hearing loss.*
2. *Auditory deprivation in the left ear may account for significant decrease in word recognition as a*

PART 3   Audiological Diagnosis and Management of Hearing Loss in the Older Adult Population

result of not using amplification in that ear for the last three years.

3. • Amplification for the left ear, which may reverse auditory deprivation in that ear.
   • Auditory training.
   • Communication strategies training to improve communication skills.

PATIENT 8

1. SRT was 35 dB HL in the right ear and 45 dB HL in the left ear. Word recognition results obtained at 40 dB SL re: SRT were 72% in the right ear and 76% in the left ear. Tympanograms suggested normal middle-ear pressure with normal tympanic membrane mobility. Contralateral acoustic reflexes were elicited within expected levels and were not measurable at 4000 Hz bilaterally. Acoustic reflex decay was negative at 500 Hz and 1000 Hz bilaterally.

2. He could not participate due to cognitive status and inability to respond consistently.

3. DPOAEs in each ear.

4. • Hard-wire assistive listening system or FM system would be the best choice for this patient due to his cognitive deficits.
   • Referral for neuropsychological evaluation to assess cognitive status. Patient should be evaluated using assistive listening device.

5. • Discussion of the relationship between hearing loss and cognition.
   • Demonstration of how to use the assistive listening device.
   • Address how to ensure that the device does not get lost on damaged.
   • Effective communication strategies to improve J.S.'s overall communication skills.

PATIENT 9

1. Sensorineural

2. • Moderate-to-profound sensorineural hearing loss.
   • Normal middle-ear functioning bilaterally.
   • Fair word recognition ability at 40 dB SL re: SRT.

3.

4. • Audiological monitoring of hearing sensitivity as Lyme disease progresses.
   • Balance evaluation and possible rehabilitation depending on the findings and symptoms.
   • Amplification selection and fitting.
   • Communication strategies training to improve communication skills.

PATIENT 10

1. One area of concern is the asymmetry of the sensorineural hearing loss in the high frequencies (4000–8000 Hz), with the right ear being significantly poorer.

   A second concern is the asymmetrical word recognition score at 40 dB SL, with right ear performance classified as poor and left ear classified as excellent. Rollover is present in the right ear, which suggests retrocochlear involvement.

   A third concern is the presence of acoustic reflex decay at 500 Hz and 1000 Hz in the right ear, which suggests retrocochlear involvement.

   The absolute and interpeak latencies for the ABR were normal in the left ear. No waves were present in the right ear.

2. A possible etiology is an VIII nerve tumor.

3. • Referral to a neurotologist for medical evaluation and MRI.
   • Audiological follow-up as necessary to monitor hearing.

References

Abrams, W., Beers, M., & Berkow, R. (1995). *The Merck manual of geriatrics* (2nd ed.). Whitehouse Station, NJ: Merck.

Ballachandra, B. B. (1995). *The human ear canal: Theoretical considerations and clinical applications including cerumen management.* San Diego: Singular.

Bess, F., Lechentenstein, M., Logan, S., Burger, M., & Nelson, E. (1989). Hearing impairment as a determinant of function in the elderly. *Journal of the American Geriatrics Society, 37*, 123–128.

Botwinick, J. (1970). *Aging and behavior.* New York: Springer.

Busacco, D. (2009). Make your practice accessible for patients with dual sensory loss. *Advance for Audiologists, 11*(3), 50–53.

Cooper, J. (1994). Health and Nutrition Examination Survey of 1971–75. Part 1: Ear and race effects in hearing. *Journal of the American Academy of Audiology, 5*, 30–36.

DeWane, J. A. (1995). Dealing with dizziness and disequilibrium in older patients: A clinical approach. *Geriatric Rehabilitation, 11*, 30–38.

Gates, G., Cobb, J., Linn, R., Rees, T., Wolf, P., & D'Agostino, R. (1996). Central auditory dysfunction, cognitive dysfunction and dementia in older people. *Archives of Otolaryngology Head and Neck Surgery, 122*, 161–167.

Gordin-Salant, S. (1987). Age-related differences in speech recognition as a function of test format and paradigm. *Ear and Hearing, 8*, 277–282.

Gorga, M., Neeley, S., Ohlrich, B., Hoover, B., Redner, J., & Peters, J. (1997). From laboratory to clinic: A large scale study of distortion product otoacoustic emissions in ears with normal hearing and ears with hearing loss. *Ear and Hearing, 18*, 440–455.

Hall, J. (2007). *New handbook of auditory evoked responses.* Boston: Allyn & Bacon.

Harris, F., & Probst, R. (1997). Otoacoustic emissions and audiometric outcomes. In M. Robinette & T. Glattke (Eds.), *Otoacoustic emissions—clinical applications* (pp. 213–242). New York: Thieme Medical.

Hollowich, F. (1985). *Ophthalmology* (2nd ed.). New York: Thieme-Stratton.

Hull, R. (2004). *Aural rehabilitation.* San Diego: Singular.

Jacobson, G., Newman G., & Kartush, J. (1997). *Handbook of balance function testing.* San Diego: Singular.

Jerger, J., Silman, S., Lew, H. L. & Chmiel, M. (1993). Case studies in binaural interference: Converging evidence from behavioral and electrophysiological measurements. *Journal of the American Academy of Audiology, 7,* 406–418.

Lansbury-Martin, B., Martin, G., & Whitehead, M. (1997). Distorion product otoacoustic emissions. In M. Robinette & T. Glattke (Eds.), *Otoacoustic emissions—Clinical applications* (pp. 116–142). New York: Thieme Medical.

Katz, J. (Ed). (2002). *Handbook of clinical audiology* (5th ed.). Baltimore: Lippincott Williams & Wilkins.

Kricos, P. (2007). Hearing assistive technology considerations for older individuals with dual sensory loss. *Trends in amplification, 11,* 273–279.

Mulrow, C., Agular, C., Endicott, G., & Tuley, M. (1990). Quality of life changes and hearing impairment results of randomized trail. *Annals of Internal Medicine, 113,* 188–194.

Musiek, F. E., & Geurhink, N. A. (1981). Auditory brainstem and middle latency evoked response sensitivity hear threshold. *Annals of Otology, Rhinology and Laryngology, 90,* 236–240.

National Council on Aging. (1999). The consequence of untreated hearing loss in older persons. Retrieved from http://www.ncoa.org

Pfeiffer, E. (1975). A short-portable mental status questionnaire for the assessment of organic brain deficit in elderly patients. *Journal of the American Geriatrics Society, 23,* 433–441.

Stach, B. (1999). *Clinical audiology: An introduction.* San Diego: Singular.

Tychin, S. (1997). Coping with hearing loss. *Seminars in Hearing, 18,* 77–86.

Uhlmann, R., Larson, E., Rees, T., Koepsell, T., & Duckert, L. (1989). Relationship of hearing impairment to dementia and cognitive dysfunction in older adults. *Journal of the American Medical Association, 261*(13), 1916–1919.

Walden, T., & Walden, B. (2005). Unilateral versus bilateral amplification for adults with impaired hearing. *Journal of the American Academy of Audiology, 16*(8), 574–584.

Weinstein, B. (2000). *Geratric audiology.* New York: Thieme.

Weinstein, B., & Amsel, L. (1986). Hearing loss and senile dementia in the institutionalized elderly. *Clinical Gerontologist, 4,* 3–15.

Weinstein, B., & Ventry, I. (1983). Audiometric correlates of the Hearing Handicap Inventory for the Elderly. *Journal of Speech and Hearing Disorders, 48,* 379–384.

Recommended Readings

American Speech-Language-Hearing Association (ASHA). (1997). Guidelines for audiology service delivery in nursing home. *American Speech-Language-Hearing Association*, 29(Suppl. 17), 15–29.

Chmiel, R., & Jerger, J. (1996). Hearing aid use, central auditory disorder and hearing handicap in elderly persons. *Journal of the American Academy of Audiology, 7*, 190–202.

Chmiel, R., Jerger, J., Murphy, E. Pirozzolo, F., & Tooley-Young, C. (1997). Unsuccessful use of binaural amplification by an elderly person. *Journal of the American Academy of Audiology, 8*(1), 1–10.

Dubno, J., Dirko, D., & Morgan, D. (1984). Effects of age and mild hearing loss on speech recognition in noise. *Journal of the Acoustical Society of America, 76*, 87–96.

Gordin-Salant, S., & Fitzgerald, P. (1993). Temporal factors and speech recognition performance in young and elderly listeners. *Journal Speech and Hearing Research, 36*, 1276–1285.

Jackson, L. (2005). Lyme disease and hearing loss. *Audiology Online*. Retrieved May 10, 2009, from http://www.audiologyonline.com/askexpert/display_question.asp?question_id=325

Jerger, J., Jerger, S., Oliver, T., & Pirozzolo, F. (1989). Speech understanding in the elderly. *Ear and Hearing, 10*, 79–89.

Kemp, D. (1978). Simulated acoustic emissions within the human auditory system. *Journal of the Acoustical Society, 64*, 1386–1391.

Marshall, L. (1981). Auditory processing in aging listeners. *Journal of Speech and Hearing Disorders, 46*, 226–240.

National Council on Aging. (1999). The consequences of untreated hearing loss in older persons. Retrieved May 10, 2009, from http://www.ncoa.org

Palmer, C., Adams, S., Bourgeous, M., Durrant, J., & Rossi, M. (1999). Reduction in caregiver-identified problem behaviors in patients with Alzheimer's disease post-hearing aid fitting. *Journal of Speech-Language-Hearing Research, 42*, 312–328.

Salthouse, T., & Davis, H. (2006). Organization of cognitive abilities and neuropsychological variables across the lifespan. *Developmental Review, 26,* 31–54.

Schuknecht, H., & Gacek, M. (1993). Cochlear pathology in presbycusis. *Annals of Oto-Rhino-Laryngology, 102,* 1–16.

Silman, S., Silverman, C., Emmer, M., & Gelfand, S. (1992). Adult-onset auditory deprivation. *Journal of the American Academy of Audiology, 3,* 390–396.

Silverman, C. A., & Silman, S. (1990). Apparent auditory deprivation from monaural amplification and recovery with binaural amplification. *Journal of the American Academy of Audiology, 1,* 175–180.

Stach, B. A., Loiselle, L. H., & Jerger, J. (1991). Special hearing aid considerations in elderly persons with auditory processing disorders. *Ear & Hearing, 12*(Suppl. 6), 131–138.

Stover, L., & Norton, S. (1993). The effects of aging on otoacoustic emissions. *Journal of the Acoustical Society of America, 94,* 2670–2681.

Vaughan, N., & Fausti, S. (2006). *The aging auditory system: Considerations for rehabilitation.* Proceedings from the National Center for Rehabilitative Auditory Research, 2005 Portland, OR. New York: Thieme.

Weinstein, B., & Amsel, L. (1986). Hearing loss and senile dementia in the institutionalized elderly. *Clinical Gerontologist, 4,* 3–15.

Glossary

Absolute wave latency   The time in msec that each of the auditory-evoked potential wavelengths appear after acoustic stimulation.

Acoustic admittance   Amount of energy that flows through the middle ear.

Acoustic reflex   Contraction of the tensor tympani and stapedius muscles of the middle ear in response to loud sounds. It is thought that these muscles protect the ear from damage due to intense acoustic stimulation.

Acoustic reflex decay   Decrease in the magnitude of the acoustic reflex by 50% or greater from the onset of the response.

Acoustic reflex threshold   The lowest intensity that produces an acoustic reflex.

Air-bone gap   The amount in dB that air conduction exceeds bone conduction at a particular frequency.

Air conduction   Hearing sensitivity measured from the outer ear to the inner ear.

Asymmetrical hearing loss   Hearing loss that is greater in one ear by 20 dB HL or more.

Attention-deficit/hyperactivity disorder   A neurological condition that involves difficulty with attention and possible auditory processing involvement.

Audiogram   Graphic representation of hearing sensitivity as a function of intensity and frequency.

Audiologic rehabilitation   Management of hearing loss using a variety of techniques including amplification, auditory training, speechreading, counseling, and/or communication strategies to maximize residual hearing.

Audiologist   Master or doctorate-level professional who specializes in the diagnosis and rehabilitation of hearing and balance disorders.

Audiometer   Electrical instrument, either manual or computerized, used to assess hearing sensitivity.

Audiometric zero   Average normal hearing thresholds for a range of frequencies tested.

Auditory brainstem response   Objective measurement of the integrity of the auditory system from VIII nerve to the brainstem, designated by waveforms I, II, III, IV, V, VI, and VII. These waveforms are present within 7 msec following high-intensity acoustic stimulation.

Auditory-evoked potentials   Electrical responses recorded using electrodes placed on the scalp. These potentials are defined based on the latency at which they occur after acoustic stimulation. The time at which they occur is related to their location from VIII nerve to the auditory cortex.

Auditory neuropathy   Normal hearing or no greater than moderate sensorineural hearing loss with poorer speech understanding ability and presence of OAEs but absence of ABR results.

Auditory processing disorder   Difficulty in perceptual processing of auditory information in the central nervous system that can cause problems with speech understanding.

Barotrauma   Damage to the ear due to sudden fluctuation in air pressure that can occur when diving or flying.

Behavioral observation audiometry (BOA)   The audiologist observes a patient's behavior in response to the presence or absence of acoustic stimuli.

Bilateral   Hearing with two ears.

Binaural   Listening with two ears.

Bone-anchored hearing aid   Hearing aid implanted into the middle ear; commonly recommended in cases of outer and/or middle ear disorders such as atresia or chronic otitis media.

Bone conduction   Promulgation of sound by direct transfer of vibrations of the bones of the skull to the inner ear.

Cochlear implant   Typically recommended in cases of severe-to-profound hearing loss with limited or no benefit from amplification. It consists of internal components including a receiver and electrodes that are implanted into the inner ear. The external components include a microphone and signal processor.

Collapsed ear canal   Temporary conductive hearing loss due to the pressure from supra-aural earphones that cause the external auditory canal to close. This condition is common in the pediatric and geriatric populations. Once the earphones are removed the conductive hearing loss is ameliorated.

Conductive hearing loss   Hearing loss due to damage to the outer and/or middle ear.

Cross-hearing   Perception of sound as a result of the test stimulus being heard in the nontest ear.

Deaf   Individuals with a severe-to-profound hearing loss who receive minimal benefit from hearing aids. Oftentimes, an alternative mode of communication such as American Sign Language (ASL) is used for communication.

Dementia   Anatomical changes in the brain related to aging, resulting in reduced memory capacity that can range from mild to severe.

Distortion-product otoacoustic emissions (DPOAEs)   Nonlinear process in the cochlea resulting from stimulation of the outer hair cells. Two tones, f_1 and f_2, are presented with the most robust DPOAE present at the frequency resulting from $2f_1-f_2$. Provides information about the intactness of the outer hair cells.

Effective masking   Amount of threshold shift yielded by a given level of noise to eliminate cross-hearing so that the nontest ear cannot participate in the hearing assessment.

False negative response   Failure to respond to acoustic stimuli.

False positive response   Response to an acoustic stimulus when no sound is present.

Frequency   Number of oscillations per second as measured in Hertz (Hz).

Functional hearing loss   Exaggeration of hearing threshold levels.

Genetic counseling   Counseling regarding the possibility of a genetic condition and the likelihood of passing the condition to future generations (e.g., hearing loss).

Habituation   Reduction in behavioral responses over time in infants and young children during subjective audiological tests such as behavioral observation audiometry.

Hard of hearing   Minimal to severe hearing loss. Typically, individuals use amplification effectively and benefit from a variety of audiologic rehabilitation techniques to maximize residual hearing.

Hearing aid   Amplification device that can be digital or analog. A variety of styles and electroacoustic characteristics are available.

Hearing handicap   Self-perception of the impact of hearing loss on one's daily lifestyle, assessed using hearing handicap and communication scales.

Hearing level (HL)   Lowest intensity at which sound is detectable.

Impedance   Resistance to the flow of energy.

Insert earphones   Earphones that are inserted into the external auditory canal. Their advantages include increased patient comfort, reduction of ambient noise, elimination of collapsed canals, and higher levels of interaural attenuation, which reduces the need for masking.

Intensity   Amount of sound energy measured in decibels (dB).

Interaural attenuation   Reduction in the intensity of sound as it travels via bone conduction from one side of the head to the opposite side.

Interpeak wave latency   The amount of time in msec between two waves of the ABR; typically measure waves I–III, III–IV, and I–V.

Localization Ability to determine the location or direction of a sound source.

Loudness discomfort level (LDL) Level of acoustic stimuli that is uncomfortable to listen to for an extended period of time.

Masking Introduction of noise to one ear through an earphone to eliminate the nontest ear from hearing and participating in the test situation.

Maximum masking level Maximum amount of noise that can be used before the noise can cross over to the test ear and shift the hearing threshold level to eliminate cross-hearing.

Ménière's disease Inner-ear condition that causes tinnitus, fluctuating hearing loss, vertigo, and nausea and/or vomiting.

Mental retardation Lower-than-normal intelligence, falling below 100 Intelligence Quotient (I.Q).

Middle latency response Auditory potentials that occur 10 msec to 50 msec after stimulus onset.

Minimum masking level Amount of noise that can cause a threshold shift in the nontest ear to eliminate it from participating in the test situation.

Mixed hearing loss Result of damage to the outer and/or middle ear and inner ear.

Monaural Listening with one ear.

Most comfortable listening Hearing level for acoustic stimuli that is identified as most comfortable to listen to over a period of time.

Multiple sclerosis Progressive neurological condition that result in demyelization of the nervous system, which may result in a sensorineural hearing loss.

Narrowband noise Noise that is passed through a band-pass filter that is centered around an audiometric frequency.

Neonatal intensive care unit Intensive care unit specifically for newborns with significant medical conditions.

Noise-induced hearing loss Caused by exposure to loud noise either on a one-time basis, referred to as an acoustic trauma, or by exposure over time resulting in a permanent threshold shift causing a sensorineural hearing loss.

NU-CHIPS Picture identification test for young children to assess word recognition abilities; standardized on children with hearing loss.

Occlusion effect The increase in loudness of a tone presented via bone conduction when the outer ear is covered with an earphone for masking purposes.

Otitis media Fluid in the middle-ear space that can result in a conductive hearing loss. May be treated with antibiotics and/or pressure equalization (P.E.) tubes.

Otoacoustic emissions Sounds emanating from the cochlea that are picked up by a probe tube microphone placed in the external auditory canal.

Otosclerosis   Middle-ear condition in which spongy, bony growth surrounds the stapes footplate and the cochlea.

Otoscope   Light device that can be use to visually inspect the outer ear.

Ototoxic   Toxic to the auditory and/or vestibular system.

Overmasking   The phenomenon that results when the masking noise presented to the nontest ear is so intense that due to cross-hearing it is heard in the test ear along with the acoustic stimulus.

PB Maximum (PB Max)   Highest score for phonetically balanced (PB) words obtained during speech recognition testing.

Performance intensity function   A graph that demonstrates word recognition score as a function of intensity or presentation level.

Peripheral hearing loss   Hearing loss that can involve the outer, middle, and/or inner ear.

Pervasive developmental disorder   Spectrum of autism disorders that result in social, cognitive, and communication disorders.

Phonetically balanced (PB) word lists   Word lists that contain speech sounds that typically occur with the same frequency as in everyday conversational speech. Commonly used PB word lists include those by Northwest University (i.e., NU#6) and Central Institute for the Deaf (i.e., CID W-22).

Pressure equalization (P.E.) tube   Small ventilation tube placed in the tympanic membrane that allows for air pressure to enter the middle-ear space.

Pure tone audiometry   Assessment of pure tone thresholds for air and bone conduction to determine the type, degree, and audiometric configuration of the hearing loss.

Pure tone average (PTA)   Average of the pure tone air conduction thresholds calculated at 500 Hz, 1000 Hz, and 2000 Hz in each ear.

Pure tone threshold   Lowest intensity level at which a pure tone can be heard 50% of the time.

Reliability   Consistency of responses over time.

Residual hearing   Amount of useable hearing.

Retrocochlear hearing Loss   Hearing loss due to pathology involving the VIII nerve.

Rollover ratio   Defined as the maximum score minus the minimum score over the maximum score. The score provides information about the integrity of the VIII nerve. If the ratio is .45 or greater, then rollover is present, which suggests VIII nerve pathology.

Sensorineural hearing loss   Hearing loss due to damage to the cochlea and/or VIII nerve.

Site of lesion   Location of pathology in the ear.

Sound level meter   Allows for the measurement of the intensity of sound.

Speech audiometry   Battery of tests to assess the ability to understand speech in a variety of listening conditions, such as quiet and noise.

Speech noise   Filtering of white noise above 1000 Hz at a rate of 12 dB per octave.

Speech reception threshold/speech recognition threshold/spondee threshold   Lowest intensity in which 50% of spondee words are repeated correctly.

Spondee   Two-syllable word with equal stress on each syllable.

Spontaneous otoacoustic emissions   Otoascoustic emissions that are present in the outer ear without any eliciting auditory signal.

Stenger test   Can be done for pure tone or speech stimuli to assess for the presence of functional hearing loss. The test will be positive, meaning functional loss is present, or negative, meaning it is not present.

Supra-aural earphones   Earphones and cushions mounted in a large cup that cover the pinna, designed to attenuate background noise.

Symmetrical hearing loss   Degree of hearing loss that is equal in both ears.

Tinnitus   Ringing, buzzing, or some other auditory sensation in the ear(s) and or head.

Transient-evoked otoacoustic emissions (TEOAEs)   Otoacoustic emissions elicited by a transient auditory signal such as a click. They are present between 4 and 10 msec following stimulus presentation and provide information on the integrity of the outer hair cells in the cochlea.

Tympanogram   Graph that illustrates the pressure-compliance function as air pressure is varied in the external auditory canal.

Tympanometry   Measurement of the compliance of the tympanic membrane as a function of varying air pressure in the ear canal.

Undermasking   This phenomenon results when the masking noise presented to the nontest ear is not of sufficient intensity to prevent cross-hearing to the nontest ear.

Unilateral   Hearing in one ear.

Validity   Truth of a response.

Vertigo   Sensation of spinning or whirling of a person or the environment. Subjective vertigo is when the person seems to be spinning or whirling. Objective vertigo is the perception of the environment spinning or whirling.

Word recognition score   Maximum percentage score obtained for word stimuli, with 100% presented at a loud level being the maximum score and 0% the minimum score. The higher the score, the better the person's speech understanding abilities.

Index

Acoustic immittance battery, 27–31
  acoustic reflex decay, 31
  acoustic reflex thresholds, 30–31
  static acoustic compliance, 29–30
  tympanometry, 27–29
Acoustic reflex decay, 31
Acoustic reflex thresholds, 30–31
Activities of daily living (ADL), 130, 139
  cognition and, 133
Adults, classification of hearing loss in, 4
Aging. *See also* Older adult population
  audiometric testing and, 135
  auditory brainstem response and, 136
  auditory late responses and, 136
  biological changes in, 131–35
  impacts of, 135–36
  middle latency response and, 136
  otoacoustic emissions and, 135–36
  psychosocial issues related to, 136–37
  speech perception and, 135
American National Standards Institute (ANSI),
  Standards for Allowable Ambient Noise
  Levels, 14
American Speech-Language-Hearing
  Association (ASHA)
  case history, 8–9
  sample audiogram from, 9, 10
Americans with Disabilities Act (ADA), 74
Amplification devices, for children, 91
Attention-deficit/hyperactivity disorder
  (ADHD), 88
Audiogram, recording speech audiometry
  results on, 26
Audiogram interpretation, 1–34
  answers to exercises, 65–68, 121–23, 165–67
  exercises, 35–62, 93–117, 141–62
Audiological data, recording, 33–34
Audiological diagnosis, in older adult
  population, 129–63
Audiological evaluation, of nursing home
  residents, 137
Audiological rehabilitation, in older adults
  auditory status and, 139
  cognition and, 139
  manual dexterity and, 139
  psychological status and, 139–40
  visual status and, 138
Audiologic diagnosis, in children, 73–127
Audiologic evaluation, components of, 6–8
  case history interview, 6–7, 8–9
  otoscopic evaluation, 7
Audiologic intervention, for children with
  hearing loss, 90–92
Audiometric configuration, 5
  classification of, 5
Audiometric testing, impacts of aging on, 135

Audiometric testing principles, 1–34
Auditory brainstem response (ABR), 27, 32–33
  impact of aging on, 136
  testing in children, 85–86
Auditory evoked potentials (AEP), 18, 27
Auditory late responses (ALR), impact of aging
  on, 136
Auditory neuropathy, in children, 89
Auditory processing disorders (APD), 2, 87, 139
  attention-decifit/hyperactivity disorder and, 88
  in children, 88
Auditory system
  changes in, 134–35
  objective assessment of, 26–33
Augmentative and alternative communication
  (AAC) devices, 16

Behavioral observation audiometry (BOA), 80
Behavioral testing, of children, 77–81
  behavioral observation audiometry, 80
  conditioned orientation reflex audiometry, 81
  conditioned play audiometry, 81
  visual reinforcement audiometry, 80–81
Behind-the-ear (BTE) digital programmable
  hearing aids, 90–91
Biological changes, in aging, 131–35
  auditory system, 134–35
  cardiovascular system, 132
  cognition, 133
  immune system, 132–33
  nervous system, 131
  renal system, 132
  somatosensory system, 133
  vestibular system, 133–34
  visual system, 132
Bone-anchored hearing aid (BAHA), 87
Bone conduction audiometry, 9–19

Cardiovascular system, changes in, 132
Carrier phrase, 23–24
Case history interview, 6–7, 8–9
  ASHA, 8–9
  pediatric, 77, 78–79
Cerumen, impacted, 16–17
Children
  amplification devices for, 90–91
  attention-decifit/hyperactivity disorder in, 88
  audiogram interpretation exercises, 93–117
  audiologic assessment in, 76–86
  audiologic diagnosis in, 73–127
  audiologic intervention for, 90–92
  auditory neuropathy in, 88–89
  auditory processing disorders in, 88
  behavioral testing of, 77–81
  classification of hearing loss in, 4
  clinical enrichment projects, 119–20

cochlear implants for, 91
early infant hearing detection programs, 75–76
educational options for, 91–92
functional hearing loss in, 89
hearing loss management in, 73–127
impacted cerumen in, 17
intervention with culturally and linguistically
  diverse, 90
masking in, 86
objective testing of, 83–86
otitis media in, 86–87
with physical and mental challenges, 89–90
special considerations in, 86–90
speech audiometry testing in, 82–83
testing guidelines for, 73–75
unilateral hearing loss in, 87–88
Clinical enrichment projects
  for audiogram interpretation, 63–64
  for children, 119–20
  for older adult population, 163
Cochlear implants, for children, 91
Cognition, changes in, 133
Cognitive impairment, audiologic evaluation of
  older adults with, 138
Completely-in-the-canals (CIC), 134
Conditioned orientation reflex (COR)
  audiometry, 81, 89
Conductive hearing loss, 3, 30, 33
Cross-hearing, 11
Culturally diverse patients
  intervention with, 90
  testing, 26

Dementia, 133
Demographics, of older adults in United States,
  130–31
Difficult-to-test patients, in pure tone
  audiometry, 18
Distortion product otoacoustic emissions
  (DPOAE), 31, 85, 136

Ear canals, collapsed, 15
Early Hearing Detection and Intervention
  (EDHI), 75
Early infant hearing detection programs, 75–76
Earphone selection, 15
Educational options, for children, 91–92
Effective masking (EM), 12
Electronystagmography (ENG), 134
English as a second language (ESL), 6

Federal Education of the Handicapped Act, 76
Fetal alcohol syndrome, 85
Fletcher's Average, 11
Functional hearing loss, 4, 18–19
  in children, 89

Habituation, 80
Hearing Handicap Inventory for the Elderly
    (HHIE), 137
Hearing in Noise Test (HINT), 21
Hearing loss
    acoustic reflex thresholds and, 30–31
    in children, 90–92
    conductive, 3, 30
    degree of, 4–5
    functional, 4, 18–19
    mixed, 3–4
    in older adult population, 129–63
    overview of, 2–5
    in pediatric population, 73–127
    population demographics and, 1–2
    retrocochlear, 33
    sensorineural, 3
    sensorineural-cochlear, 30
    sensorineural-retrocochlear, 31
    types of, 3–4

Immittance testing, in children, 84–85
Immune system, changes in, 132–33
Impacted cerumen, in pure tone audiometry,
    16–17
Inconsistent responses, in pure tone
    audiometry, 16
Individualized Education Plan (IEP), 74
Individualized Family Service Plan (IFSP), 74,
    76

Joint Committee on Infant Hearing (JCIH), 75

Loudness discomfort level (LDL), 22, 26
Loudness level, in speech audiometry, 21–22

Malingering hearing loss. *See* Functional
    hearing loss
Masking
    in children, 86
    effective, 12
    problems, 14
    for pure tone air conduction, 12–13
    for pure tone audiometry, 11–14
    for pure tone bone conduction, 13
    for speech audiometry, 22–23
Mental Status Questionnaire (MSQ), 138
Middle latency response (MLR), 33
    impact of aging on, 136
Minimum levels of response (MLR), 80
Mixed hearing loss, 3–4
Monosyllabic-Trochee-Spondee Test (MST), 83
Moro Reflex, 80
Most comfortable listening level (MCL), 20, 21,
    26

Nervous systems, changes in, 131
Nonorganic hearing loss. *See* Functional
    hearing loss
*Northwestern University Children With Hearing
    Impairment (NU-CHIPS)*, 83

Objective testing, of pediatric population,
    83–86

auditory brainstem response testing, 85–86
immittance testing, 84–85
otoacoustic emissions testing, 85
Older adult population. *See also* Aging
    audiogram interpretation exercises, 141–62
    audiological diagnosis and hearing loss
        management, 129–63
    audiological rehabilitation considerations in,
        138–40
    biological changes in, 131–35
    clinical enrichment projects, 163
    with cognitive impairment, 138
    demographics of, 130–31
    guidelines for testing, 129–30
    in nursing homes, 137
    psychosocial issues in, 136–37
    special considerations in testing, 137–38
Otitis media, in children, 86–87
Otoacoustic emissions (OAE), 31–32, 75, 89, 90
    impact of aging on, 135–36
    testing in children, 85
Otoscopic evaluation, 7
Overmasking, 14

Pediatric audiologic assessment, 76–86
    behavioral testing and, 77–81
    case history interview, 77, 78–79
Phonetically Balanced Kindergarten (PB-K)
    word lists, 83
Phonetically Balanced Performance Intensity
    (PB-PI) function, 20
Presbycusis, 134
Pressure equalization (PE) tubes, 84
Pure tone air, 9–19
Pure tone air conduction
    masking for, 12–13
Pure tone audiometry
    collapsed ear canals, 15
    difficult-to-test patients, 18
    earphone selection, 15
    impacted cerumen, 16–17
    inconsistent responses, 16
    principles of masking for, 11–14
    recording results, 14
    response mode, 15–16
    tactile responses, 16
    test environment, 14
    test instructions, 15
    tinnitus interference, 17–18
Pure tone average (PTA), 5, 11, 16, 18
Pure tone bone conduction, masking for, 13

Quick Speech in Noise Test (Quick SIN), 21, 139

Renal system, changes in, 132
Response mode, for pure tone audiometry,
    15–16
Retrocochlear hearing loss, 33

Sensorineural-cochlear hearing loss, 30
Sensorineural hearing loss, 3, 33
Sensorineural-retrocochlear hearing loss, 31
Somatosensory system, changes in, 133
Soundfield speech audiometry, 25–26

Speech audiometry, 19–26
    issues in, 23–25
    loudness level, 21–22
    masking for, 22–23
    recording results on audiogram, 26
    soundfield, 25–26
    speech detection threshold/speech awareness
        threshold, 20
    speech recognition threshold/speech
        reception threshold, 19
    testing culturally and linguistically diverse
        patients, 26
    word recognition score, 20–21
Speech audiometry testing, in children, 82–83
    speech detection/speech awareness threshold,
        82
    speech reception threshold testing, 82
    word recognition testing, 82–83
Speech awareness threshold (SAT), 20, 26
Speech detection threshold/speech awareness
    threshold, 20
    in children, 82
Speech perception, impact of aging on, 135
Speech Perception in Noise (SPIN), 21
Speech recognition threshold/speech reception
    threshold, 19
Speech recognition threshold (SRT), 16, 18
Staggered Spondaic Word (SSW), 21
Standards for Allowable Ambient Noise Levels
    (ANSI), 14
Static acoustic compliance, 29–30
Stenger Test, 18
Synthetic Sentence Identification (SSI), 21

Tactile responses, in pure tone audiometry, 16
Test environment
    for pure tone audiometry, 14
    for speech audiometry, 23
Testing guidelines, pediatric, 73–75
Test instructions, for pure tone audiometry, 15
Tinnitus, 3
Tinnitus interference, in pure tone audiometry,
    17–18
Transient evoked otoacoustic emissions
    (TEOAE), 31, 135
Tympanometry, 27–29

Uncomfortable listening level (UCL), 22, 26
Undermasking, 14
Unilateral hearing loss, in children, 87–88
United States
    demographics of older adults in, 130–31
    hearing loss in, 1–2

Vestibular system, changes in, 133–34
Visual reinforcement audiometry (VRA),
    80–81, 89
Visual system, changes in, 132

*Word Intelligibility by Picture Identification
    (WIPI)*, 83
Word recognition score, in speech audiometry,
    20–21
Word recognition testing, in children, 82–83